TRIAL BY FIRE

Lessons from the History of Clinical Trials

What can we learn from the past that may be relevant to modern clinical research?

In this book Dr Allan Gaw draws on the experience of two decades working in clinical trials to show how the past can illuminate the present and help us understand our current position.

In a series of intriguing stories that take us from Babylon and Ancient Egypt, to Europe in the 17th and 18th Centuries, and on to the concentration camps of Nazi Germany, and the US in the 60s and 70s, he demonstrates the origins of randomisation and blinding in clinical trials; the importance of consent, trust and codes of ethical practice; and the crucial importance of publication. And he shows us where it may have all begun.

Allan Gaw, MD, PhD, FRCPath, FFPM is Director of Operations at the Glasgow Clinical Research Facility. He is the author or editor of 14 books mostly on the subjects of Clinical Biochemistry, Cardiovascular Research, and Lipid Metabolism. You can learn more about him and his work at www.allangaw.com

OTHER WORKS BY THE AUTHOR

Gaw A and Shepherd J *Coronary Risk Factors Measurement and Management*. Martin Dunitz, London, 1999.

Gaw A and Shepherd J (eds) *Atherosclerosis and Lipid Annual 2001*. Martin Dunitz, London, 2001.

Gaw A *Statins in General Practice* 2nd edition Martin Dunitz, London, 2003.

Gaw A and Shepherd J *Statins and Stroke Prevention*, Science Press, Tokyo, 2003.

Gaw A and Shepherd J (eds) *Atherosclerosis and Lipid Annual 2003*, Martin Dunitz, Taylor Francis Group, London, 2003.

Gaw A, Packard CJ and Shepherd J (eds) *Statins: the HMG CoA reductase inhibitors in perspective*, 2nd edition, Martin Dunitz, London, 2004.

Lindsay GM and Gaw A (eds) *Coronary Heart Disease Prevention: A Handbook for the Health-care Team* 2nd edition, Harcourt Brace, Edinburgh, 2004.

Gaw A, Murphy MA, Cowan RA, O'Reilly D St J, Stewart MJ and Shepherd J: *Clinical Biochemistry An Illustrated Colour Text*. 4th edition, Elsevier, Edinburgh, 2008.

TRIAL BY FIRE

Lessons from the History of Clinical Trials

Allan Gaw

First published 2009
by SA Press

sapress42@gmail.com

Reprinted in 2012

Printed in the United Kingdom by Clydeside Press

British Library Cataloguing in Publication Data
A catalogue record for this book is available from the British
Library

ISBN 978-0-9563242-0-7

For those whose consent was never sought

CONTENTS

FOREWORD

At a celestial dinner party attended by the ancient Chinese sage Confucius, the German philosopher Friedrich Hegel, the American novelist Mark Twain, the Spanish philosopher George Santayana and the Irish dramatist Oscar Wilde, the conversation – assuming language is no barrier in heaven – may turn to history. In particular, over the port, the study of history, its purpose and its worth would be mulled over. For all these men had something profound to say about this subject and their words are as relevant today as when they were written, and especially so for the book in your hands.

This book is subtitled: "Lessons from the History of Clinical Trials". This, of course, presumes that there are indeed lessons to be learned from the study of history. Confucius certainly thinks so when he says, "Study the past if you would define the future." Santayana agrees with him. He not only values the study of history, he feels that failing to pay attention to it will have dire consequences. "Those who cannot remember the past are condemned to repeat it.", he would say. Perhaps Twain would intercede here in the conversation by agreeing that men do not necessarily learn from history, but while he declaims the actual repetition of history he does allude to the recidivism of its players, when he jokes, "The past does not repeat itself, but it rhymes." Hegel, an altogether more sober character, might bring the conversation to an abrupt close by pronouncing, "The only thing we learn from history is that we learn nothing from history."

I do not agree with Hegel, but I'm not sure I would say so to his face. It is, however, difficult to disagree with Twain. We do not always learn from history and we are sometimes condemned to relive our past mistakes. But, surely not inevitably so.

What this book is about is our need to remember the events of the past– partly to understand our present, and partly to ensure that we are forewarned of the future – a future that will "rhyme" with the past unless we pay attention to what has gone before. When I teach classes on Good Clinical Practice and Research Methods in Clinical Trials I always begin with a short history lesson. This may be seen merely as a scene setter; a way of easing into the day and a moisturizer for a rather dry subject. But, that is not why it is included. I firmly believe that unless we think about the past, analyse it and learn from it, we have little chance of really understanding what is happening now.

And what of Oscar Wilde? He is sitting uncharacteristically quietly at our dinner party. His contribution to the discussion I like to think of as the last word on the matter, especially considering a book such as this that purports to examine history and put it into a modern perspective. "[A]ny fool can make history, but it takes a genius to write it." If wishing made it so, Oscar.

Acknowledgements

This book is one of the fruits of teaching on the History of Clinical Trials for the last 6 years. As that teaching has always been as part of a team I must acknowledge the debts I owe to my colleagues and students – including Shona McDermott, Liz Tolmie, Michael Burns and especially Moira Mungall, without whose expertise and dedication our Good Clinical Practice course would not have been possible.

I would also like to thank Liz Ronald for her help in taking this manuscript from its first drafts to the finished book, and David Tolmie for his help with the cover design.

INTRODUCTION

Clinical trials are increasingly shaping modern medicine. The call to evidence based practice has never been stronger and the gold standard for that evidence is the randomised controlled clinical trial. In the field of clinical trials, as in any other human endeavour, it is always useful to look back in time in order to make sense of the world we live and work in now. By studying the past we are not only able to predict the future, but we may also understand the present.

The "present" for many conducting clinical trials is a tangled mass of bureaucracy and administrative obstacles which must be negotiated before a single patient may be seen. Frustrated by this, the commonest question I am asked by my colleagues is why is it so difficult to do a clinical trial? In order to answer this question I find myself turning to the history of my subject. By examining our history we can understand where we came from and therefore gain a better insight into how and why we have arrived at the present. Perhaps we may also use the lessons of the past to help predict what lies ahead. In short, history can be, at the very least, interesting, perhaps helpful, and maybe even much more, providing a whole contextual framework on which to hang our current and future systems of belief and practice.

In this book I wish to draw on the rich history of medicine and present a series of fascinating stories that resonate down the years and which I believe have startling relevance to our modern day practice. By thinking about our forebears and how they practiced clinical research we sometimes find ourselves holding up a mirror to ourselves.

All the examples covered in this book are taken from our Clinical Research Education and Training courses at the Glasgow Clinical Research Facility. If you would like to find out more about these courses please visit our website either at www.glasgowcrf-education.org or www.allangaw.com

There are many stories that could be retold from the history of clinical trials across the last 2,500 years. Why have I chosen the six in this book? There is a common thread that links these apparently disparate stories together. I believe they are all interesting, but more importantly they all have relevance for today. This book is not just about history – that is only the starting point – rather it is about viewing history as our tutor.

With the study of Daniel we learn the relevance and importance of publication. Without publication we would never have heard of Daniel's clinical trial. By examining the scientific endeavours of Queen Cleopatra we are reminded of the problems that any power relationship brings to the interaction between an investigator and their subjects. And, indeed, the issue of informed consent raises its head here for the first, but not the last, time in our narratives.

Van Helmont, unlike Daniel or Cleopatra, was an armchair trialist, but it is his thoughtfulness about the problems associated with investigator bias in trials that leads us to remember him and to use his story as the starting point for a discussion on the development on one of the most powerful tools in modern clinical trials – that of randomization.

If Ben Franklin had not been the American ambassador to France in 1784 we may not have had the development of trial protocols involving a blinded design, nor the introduction of placebo controls. But he was, and we do, and his story is a remarkable one. Van Helmont and Franklin both contributed in very different ways to what would now be regarded as the modern randomised controlled trial.

When we arrive at the twentieth century, and enter the uneasy realm of living memory, our stories become troubling. First we visit the US in one of its darker hours. The Tuskegee Syphilis experiment which ran from 1932-72 is now infamous and brings history up to date, for this is a story that is not shrouded in historical uncertainty in the way that our stories of Daniel and Cleopatra were. This is a story that concerned men some of whom were still alive ten years ago and whose families are still living with the consequences. Lives are changed by medical practice, and clinical trials change medical practice. But lives can also be irrevocably changed in a more direct way by medical research especially if that research is unethical. Tuskegee was such a study and its legacy for the conduct of modern clinical trials will be discussed.

Finally, we come to the concentration camps. Any discussion of the Nazi attrocities of World War II is inevitably a sombre and dispiriting affair. But, could any good come of such evil; any light from such a period of darkness? From Buchenwald to Nuremberg to the modern day clinic a clear line can be drawn. And on that line hangs the development of the codes of ethical practice that we use today and which we will explore in detail.

Of course there are many other examples we could study, and each would provide us with something unique. But the six chosen here represent some of the most important milestones in the development of the clinical trial as we understand the term today. If you are involved in any professional capacity in clinical trials, then the rich history of the subject should be a topic worthy of your study. If you are not, then clinical trials will still impact upon your life and your health, and simple curiosity to discover and understand will be sufficient reasons for reading this book.

The stories are at once fascinating and at times disturbing, but always resonant. Listen to the past – appreciate and wonder at the intelligence and ingenuity of our forebears and learn humbly from the mistakes of others.

I

DANIEL AND DIETING:

the importance of publication in clinical trials

If we think historically about clinical trials, the natural first question to ask would be: what was the first clinical trial and when did it take place? To ask this question presupposes two things. First, that in the narrative that is human history there was a time in our past before which no clinical trials had ever been performed, and after which any subsequent clinical trial could no longer claim to be the first. Second, it also presupposes that we all understand the same thing when we use the term 'clinical trial'. Although it could be argued that a slow and complex evolution of clinically related research happened over time and that the history of clinical trials is more blurred than punctuated, our first assumption, that there was at some point in history a 'first' clinical trial, seems reasonable.

However, our second assumption, presuming that the term 'clinical trial' is universally understood, is not.

Let us begin then by defining, at least for the purposes of this book, what we mean by 'clinical trial'. This is a systematic investigation designed to evaluate some form of intervention, often pharmacological, in humans. Perhaps the key word in this definition is 'systematic'. What is implied by the use of the term 'clinical trial' as opposed to an investigation, an observation or an experience is the notion of scientific rigour. When performing a clinical trial we are applying the scientific method to a clinical problem and through the study of humans and their responses to an intervention we can draw conclusions on the efficacy, safety and perhaps mode of action of that intervention.

This brings us back to the question of the first such trial. Now it is difficult, if not impossible, to know whether the evolving brains of our stone age forebears had sufficient sophistication to decide between two alternative ways of dealing with an injury based on experience. Or if, after observing that eating a particular berry led to a particular pharmacological effect like vomiting or hallucination they may not have wondered what might happen if they ate more of it or less of it. Such wonderings, if they did take place, are clearly the beginning of medical science but they can hardly be described as having advanced to the status of a clinical trial, at least by our definition above.

Over time, great civilisations have risen and fallen, and within these cultures there may have been great scientists and physicians, but without the benefit of a written record we can know nothing of the workings of their scientific minds. However, around 2600 years ago we have two contenders from Ancient Egypt and Babylon respectively. The older of the two

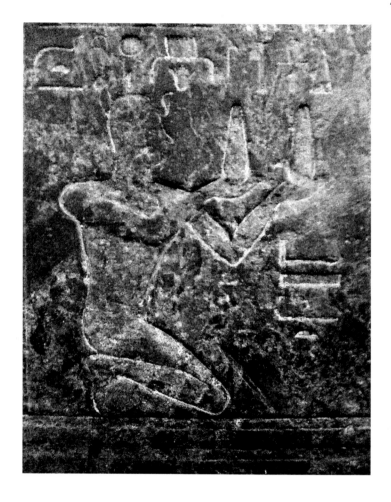

Figure 1. Basalt wall section found at Rosetta from the 26th Dynasty showing the pharaoh, Psamtek I, kneeling and making offerings to divine figures. British Museum, London (Photo by the author).

is believed to have taken place in the 7th century BCE and is recorded by the Greek historian Herodotus (1).

ANCIENT EGYPT

The pharaoh Psamtik I (also called Psammetichus), was the first of three kings of the Twenty-sixth dynasty of Egypt and reigned from 664-610 BCE (fig.1). He was interested in the origins of mankind and as Herodotus notes, "finding that mere inquiry failed to reveal which was the original race of mankind, devised an ingenious method of determining the matter." The historian goes on to describe in detail the following clinical experiment:

> "He took at random, from an ordinary family, two newly born infants and gave them to a shepherd to be brought up amongst his flocks, under strict orders that no one should utter a word in their presence...All these arrangements were made by Psammetichus because he wished to find out what word the children would first utter, once they had grown out of their meaningless baby-talk. The plan succeeded; two years later the shepherd... happened one day to open the door of the cottage and go in, when both children, running up to him with hands outstretched, pronounced the word 'becos'...Psammetichus ordered the children to be brought to him, and when he himself heard them say 'becos' he determined to find out to what language the word belonged. His inquiries revealed that it was Phrygian for 'bread', and in consideration of this the Egyptians yielded their claims and admitted the superior antiquity of the Phrygians." (1)

Herodotus goes on to relate a variation of the story whereby Psammetichus has the children raised by women whose tongues he had cut out, but he dismissed this as 'improbable'.

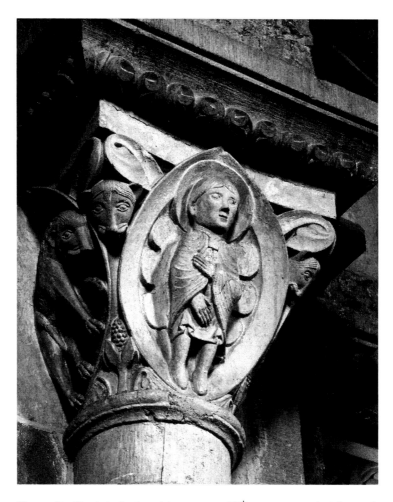

Figure 2. Daniel, depicted here on a 12th century capital from the Basilica Sainte-Marie-Madeleine de Vézelay, is more famous for his time spent in the lions' den but he may also have been the first clinical trialist.

Although this is undoubtedly a piece of clinical research, and the earlier of our two examples, we may question whether, by our definition above, it is a clinical trial at all. I would argue that it does not fulfill the necessary requirements to be regarded as a systematic investigation of an intervention. The study was non-interventional and observational.

BABYLON

In the second example we have what many would regard as the first documentary evidence of a clinical trial. In the Book of Daniel in the Old Testament, probably written sometime between the 6th and 2nd centuries BCE, we have an account of a dietary experiment in human subjects that can feasibly be regarded as the first ever documented clinical trial.

Daniel was among the many Jews who were carried off into captivity in Babylon (fig. 2). There, he and his friends were brought to work in the royal household of King Nebuchadnezzar. As part of their education and development they were required to partake of the meat and wine served in the palace, but Daniel and his friends wished to maintain their dietary independence and proposed an experiment to prove that their way was better:

> Daniel said..."Test [us] for ten days; let us be given vegetables to eat and water to drink. Then let our appearance and [that] of the youths who eat the king's rich food be observed...At the end of ten days it was seen that they were better in appearance and fatter in flesh than all the youths who ate the king's rich food." (2)

Here we have all the elements of the so-called 'modern' clinical trial. An hypothesis is postulated – in this case that what we eat and drink affects our appearance. An experiment to test this hypothesis is designed – two groups of young human subjects are given two alternative dietary regimens for 10 days. Observations are made and a conclusion is drawn – that the hypothesis is proven. Finally, and I would argue, most importantly, the findings are published – in this case in the Old Testament.

PUBLICATION

Scientific endeavour is not a private personal enterprise; it is essentially a demonstration that requires an audience for its completion. Clinical trials are scientific projects in the world of medicine and their audience may be the medical and scientific communities, the people or patients who are represented in the trial, or the lay public in general. Our first clinical trial succeeds in speaking to all these audiences, and its publication must be regarded as being in arguably the highest impact journal ever published – the Bible.

Unless we write about clinical trials and expose their findings to as wide an audience as possible we do a serious disservice to our patients and we undermine the whole purpose of our work. In this light we may ask: is the study of Daniel and his dietary trial important and worthy of a place in history because it was the first clinical trial, or does it deserve our attention because it was the first *documented* clinical trial?

As we have noted above we really have no way of ever knowing when the first investigator or team of investigators carried out the first clinical trial, if there was no written record of that project. What elevates Daniel's work to the clinical trial hall of fame is the simple fact that it was written down. This work was revealed to a wider audience, and the findings became known not just to Daniel and the people immediately involved in the study in ancient Babylon, but to countless millions across the subsequent three millennia.

From a modern perspective it may seem inconceivable that anyone or any team would go to all the trouble of conducting a clinical trial and then fail to publish their findings. But there are a number of reasons why this might be the case. Many academics find, because of the pressures on their time from teaching, administration and of course clinical duties, that writing is often low on the list of priorities. So low, on occasion, that it can drop off completely. At the other end of the spectrum there may be darker reasons why a study's results fail to see the light of day. Publication bias, whereby studies deemed to be positive are more likely to be published at all, or are published earlier and in higher impact journals, has been cited as an explanation of some of these apparently missing publications (3). Whatever the reason it has been suggested that such underreporting constitutes nothing less than scientific misconduct (4). Recently Abassi noted, "By suppressing negative findings and exaggerating positive ones, by downplaying harms and talking up benefits, healthcare decisions are based on incomplete data and ultimately harm the patients" (5)

In an attempt to correct this potential problem of missing results the International Committee of Medical Journal Editors announced in 2004 that it would only consider publication of a clinical trial if it had been registered in an appropriate registry (6). As such all clinical trials are now required to be registered in publicly accessible databases, and all investigators should ensure that the results of their completed work should be published no matter how problematic those results may be for them, their sponsors or their institutions. Good, bad or indifferent the results of a clinical trial should be made available for scrutiny.

The circle of research that begins with a question is not closed when that question is answered: it is closed when that answer is communicated to the world.

REFERENCES

1. Herodotus. The Histories, Translated by Aubrey de Sélincourt and revised by John Marincola 2003 Penguin Classics Penguin, London.
2. Daniel 1:11-16.
3. Easterbrook PJ, Berlin JA, Gopalan R, Matthews DR. Publication bias in clinical research. *Lancet* 1991; 337: 867-72.
4. Chalmers I. Underreporting research is scientific misconduct. *Journal of the American Medical Association* 1990; 263: 1405-8.
5. Abassi K. Compulsory registration of clinical trials. *British Medical Journal* 2004; 329: 637-8.
6. De Angelis C, Drazen JM, Frizelle FA, Haug C, Hoey J, Horton R et al. Clinical trials registration: a statement from the International Committee of Medical Journal Editors. *New England Journal of Medicine* 2004; 351: 1250-1.

2

CLEOPATRA AND FETAL DEVELOPMENT:

the importance of consent in clinical trials

A great deal has been written about the issue of consent in the context of clinical trials. Historically, however, this is not an issue that concerned most investigators before the 20th century. Throughout a long period the recruitment of subjects to clinical trials and their subsequent investigation, sometimes through highly invasive means, was done without any recourse to the niceties of modern medical ethical codes. Indeed, it is frankly unimaginable that many of the subjects in medical experiments throughout history would have agreed to the tests and interventions to which they were subjected if they had been asked. Although consent was a relatively alien concept in the past, it is the abuse of consent that has largely shaped our modern codes of practice. But, just how far back does it go and what can we learn from it? Perhaps the earliest documented example of such an abuse of consent takes us back just over two thousand years to the banks of the Nile and to an investigator in the unlikely form of Queen Cleopatra (fig. 3).

There were several Cleopatras in ancient Egypt, but the one that we think of when we imagine the film star Elizabeth Taylor generously endowed with eyeliner was Cleopatra the Seventh, who reigned during the 1st century BCE. History has probably been relatively unkind to this Queen of the Nile. One recent textbook described her as a "vacuous sex-kitten" (1) who conducted a series of high profile dalliances with, among others, the Romans Julius Caesar and Mark Anthony. As is often the case the reality was probably very different. Cleopatra VII was a very clever and accomplished politician, a mistress of diplomacy and probably a published scientist with a keen interest in chemistry and medicine (2). Indeed it is her venture into the field of clinical research that brings Cleopatra to our attention.

Cleopatra is reported to have devised a series of experiments to study the gestation of fetuses of different sexes. The hypothesis under test was that it took a different number of days for a male fetus and for a female fetus to develop in the uterus. To conduct her studies Cleopatra needed human subjects who she could examine at different stages of pregnancy. Examination in this case meant vivisection, and certain death both to the fetus and the mother. She chose her female servants who had been sentenced to death under government order.

These unfortunates were first forced to take medication to induce the abortion of any existing fetus. This preliminary ensured that if the handmaids were already pregnant at the time

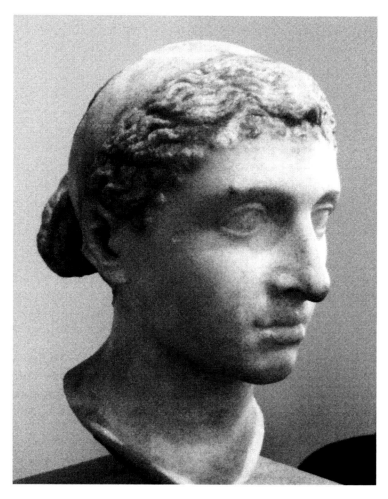

Figure 3. Cleopatra VII of Egypt 1st century BCE. Marble head, Altes Museum, Berlin.

of their sentencing their existing pregnancy would not confound the experiment.

The girls were then inseminated – the veterinary term seems appropriate – and then sacrificed for examination after varying periods of time. Their abdomens were opened and their uterine contents examined. There is little detail in the records on exactly how the examinations were conducted, but let us hope that the young women were killed humanely first.

How do we know of these experiments and did they really take place? As with much to do with Cleopatra there is a significant admixture of fact and legend in the literature. The idea that she was involved in experimental developmental biology probably comes from the writings of medieval Arabic scholars. In particular, Ibn Fatik and Ibn Usaybiah indicated that she conducted such experiments (2). Furthermore, this is taken up and discussed in Jewish Law where a discussion exists in the Babylonian Talmud on the reliability of Cleopatra's experiments and the practical significance of her results (3).

Cleopatra concluded that a male fetus was fully formed in the uterus by the 41st day of gestation, while a female fetus required 80 days to achieve completion. Of course these results were erroneous and it is interesting to speculate for a moment how such a keen and apparently rigorous scientist as Cleopatra got it so completely wrong. Most probably her attempts to ensure that at baseline the girls were all non-pregnant had failed, and may even have been confounded by the interference of the male warders put in charge of the girls to ensure their chastity before the experiments began.

What is of much greater importance, however, is the complete lack of concern shown in these studies for the well-being of the trial subjects, and the absence of any form of consent.

CONSENT

No one in Egypt at the time, nor subsequently in the medieval or renaissance worlds, nor even up to the first half of the 20th century would have contemplated seeking the consent of such trial subjects. They were nothing more than the receptacles of their investigators' reagents.

What is common to many of these studies is the power relationship that exists between investigator and subject. In the case of Cleopatra's studies the subjects were literally that, subjects of her absolute will. They were also prisoners under sentence of death and there are many instances, including some in much more recent history, where the inmates of prisons are considered fair game for eager investigators who are anxious to find a ready and unquestioning population for their studies (4). Mitford famously quoted one 20th century US investigator as saying, "Criminals in our penitentiaries are fine experimental material - and much cheaper than chimpanzees" (5).

It is easy to romanticise this piece of history. Viewed through the soft filter of 2000 years it seems so distant as to be unconnected with modern medicine and modern clinical trials. But, if this had been done within living memory would we be so forgiving? If similar experiments had been conducted in our own era on the oppressed, the incarcerated, the helpless, would we be so objective?

The medical experimentation that took place on the inmates of the Nazi concentration camps, the Japanese prisoner of war camps and indeed in prisons in the United States throughout the Second World War were really not that different to those performed by Cleopatra. Consent and its abuse were at the centre of these atrocities. No investigator sought the consent of the Jews experimented on in Dachau (6), the prisoners used for training purposes by Japanese surgeons (7), or the inmates of Stateville Prison, Illinois, who were deliberately infected with malaria (8). Consent was quite simply not a concern and was not allowed to interfere with the process of these studies. Even if it had been discussed the nature of the relationships between investigator and subject in all cases was similar to that between Cleopatra and her handmaids – one of absolute power and subjugation. It is therefore unlikely that any potential trial subject would have been in a position to refuse what was demanded of them, no matter how brutal.

That prisoners should not be used in medical research was implicit in the Nuremberg Code, but was not fully adopted by the US until 1976 (9). Despite the history of abuses and the apparently clear-cut ethical case for not using prisoners, as Cleopatra and many other investigators had done after her, a recent call was made to re-examine this question and re-open the prison doors to medical researchers (10).

When we consider the issue of *informed* consent, so central to the ethical conduct of modern day clinical trials, we take one step further away from the reality of the past. A subject cannot truly be said to have given consent if he or she does not fully understand the implications of the research and the consequences of their actions. This is a very modern concept and the nature and extent of informed consent is still being debated today (11).

What is not open to debate, however, are the core ethical principles that contain and give direction to modern clinical trials. The health and well-being of individuals prevail over any benefit to science or society and without informed consent we can, and must, do nothing (12).

CONCLUSION

It is with the goodwill and partnership of our patients that modern clinical trials move forward (13). That partnership is built on trust. That trust must be inviolable, for once it is broken it is unlikely to be repaired, and the wider damage done to medical research and eventually to clinical practice will be immeasurable.

REFERENCES

1. Bianchi RS. Cleopatra VII in The Oxford Encyclopaedia of Ancient Egypt I. Edited by Donald B. Redford. New York/Oxford. 288-291, 2001.
2. El Daly O. Egyptology: the missing millennium. Ancient Egypt in medieval Arabic writings. UCL Press 2005.
3. Babylonian Talmud, Tractate Niddah Folio 30b. http://www.come-and-hear.com/hear.com/ niddah/niddah_30.html#30b_21 (Accessed Jan 30, 2006).
4. Hornblum AM. They were cheap and available: prisoners as research subjects in twentieth century America. *British Medical Journal* 1997; 315: 1437-41.
5. Mitford J. Experiments Behind Bars: Doctors, Drug Companies, and Prisoners. *Atlantic Monthly* 23, January 1973, 64-73.
6. United States v Karl Brandt et al. Trials of war criminals. Washington DC: Government Printing Office, 1949: 9114-228.
7. Kristof, ND. Japan confronting gruesome war atrocity. *New York Times*, March 17, 1995.

8. Laurence WL. New drugs to combat malaria are tested in prisons for army. *New York Times*, March 5, 1945.

9. Government to ban medical research on federal inmates. *New York Times*, March 2, 1976.

10. Pasquerella L. Confining choices: should inmates' participation in research be limited? *Theoretical Medicine and Bioethics* 2002; 23: 519-36.

11. Flory J, Emanuel E. Interventions to improve research participants' understanding in informed consent for research: a systematic review. *Journal of the American Medical Association* 2004; 292: 1593-601.

12. ICH Harmonised Tripartite Guideline for Good Clinical Practice (GCP) http://www.ich.org/LOB/media/MEDIA482.pdf (Accessed June 17, 2009).

13. Goodare H, Lockwood S. Involving patients in clinical research. *British Medical Association* 1999; 319: 724-25.

3

VAN HELMONT AND HIS WAGER:

the importance of eliminating bias in clinical trials

When a physician has a choice of treatments for the patient sitting across her desk, what makes her choose one over the other? Is it her firm belief that one treatment is better than the other in this particular case? Is it that she has had more experience of one treatment compared to the alternative and is therefore more confident of its use? Is it simply that one treatment is newer, more interesting, or perhaps even more heavily advertised than the other? Suppose there is no rational reason at all – no legitimacy for the choice. Should we practice medicine like this? Many think we should not and have sought out ways of finding hard evidence to support our treatment decisions. They argue that if we have good, scientifically tested reasons for prescribing one treatment regimen rather than another, and we base our clinical practice on that evidence, then we are offering our patients the best medicine we can.

The best medicine then requires the best evidence and there is a consensus that this comes from the randomised controlled trial. The best modern trials have at the core of their design the notion of randomisation. This requires us to assign patients to one of two or more alternative treatment strategies, not on the basis of any particular patient characteristic such as their sex, age, or the severity of their disease, nor indeed on the basis of any physician characteristic such as experience or personal preference. Instead, we assign treatments based on chance. This is done to remove the many and varied sources of bias in the treatment decision, leaving us to test the effectiveness of the treatment alone. If the randomisation process is truly random and the study large enough we end up with virtually identical cohorts of patients that differ only in the treatment they receive. Thus, any difference in the clinical outcome of these patients over time may be assuredly ascribed to the difference in treatment alone.

Thus, the randomised controlled trial has been hailed as an innovation helping to transform modern medicine and laying the foundation stones of evidence based practice. However, to suggest that the 20th century can take the credit for this does an injustice to the past, and in particular to a Flemish physician and medicinal chemist called Jan Baptiste Van Helmont (fig. 4).

VAN HELMONT

Van Helmont was born in 1580 and was educated at Leuven. Like many young men he was unsure of which path to take in

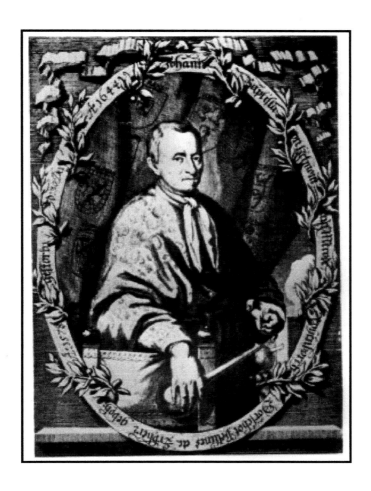

Figure 4.   Etching of Jan Baptiste Van Helmont (1580-1644).

life and studied a variety of subjects including different sciences before settling on the study of medicine.

One of his major claims to fame was his coining of the word *gas* to describe one of the states of matter. In addition, he performed experiments to demonstrate the uptake of water and air by plants. His works were collated and published in 1648, four years after his death, by his son Franciscus Mercurius Van Helmont and these works appeared in English as the *Oriatrike* in 1662 (1).

It is in this work that we find evidence of his interest in clinical trials. To settle a dispute he was having with orthodox physicians who used bloodletting and purging for treatment, Van Helmont laid the following wager:

> "Let us take out of the Hospitals, out of the Camps, or from elsewhere, 200 or 500 poor People, that have Fevers, Pleurisies etc. Let us divide them into halfes, let us cast lots, that one halfe of them may fall to my share, and the other to yours; I will cure them without bloodletting and sensible evacuation; but do you do, as ye know. . . . We shall see how many funerals both of us shall have. But let the reward of the contention or wager be, 300 florens, deposited on both sides. Here your business is decided" (1)

Whether through reticence or through ignorance, Van Helmont's wager was not accepted in his lifetime and his proposal for eliminating bias in the conduct of clinical trials slipped into obscurity for over two and half centuries.

TAKING UP THE WAGER

Van Helmont's wager was finally taken up by Amberson, McMahon and Pinner in 1931. This group assessed the effectiveness of sodium gold thiosulphate (sanocrysin) in the treatment of pulmonary tuberculosis (2). They studied 24 patients who were divided into two "matched" groups. The treatment allocation of each group was then decided by the toss of a coin as described below:

> "Obviously, the matching could not be precise, but it was as close as possible, each patient having previously been studied independently by two of us. Then, by a flip of the coin, one group became identified as group I (sanocrysin treated) and the other as group II (control)."

This was exactly the block allocation of subjects described by Van Helmont and was used as he proposed in an attempt to eliminate investigator bias in choosing which patient received which treatment.

Block allocation like this has two deficiencies as noted by Doll (3). First, it is practically almost impossible to create two matched groups, as acknowledged above by Amberson and his colleagues (2). We may match for the obvious characteristics such as age and sex and severity of disease, but there may be underlying characteristics, of which the investigator is unaware, but which may significantly affect the response of the individual patient to therapy. Second, block allocation offers no way of estimating the relevant random error.

An approach which may be seem to be one step better than block allocation is alternate allocation whereby the first patient and every odd-numbered patient thereafter receives treatment A and the second patient and every even numbered patient receives treatment B. This approach has been used for many years and significantly pre-dates many other attempts at eliminating bias.

For example, Balfour, a military physician in charge of an orphanage in which there was a Scarlet Fever outbreak, set out to evaluate the use of belladonna in the prevention of the disease in 1854 (4). His method of avoiding bias was to use an alternate allocation strategy as noted in his publication:

> "I divided [151 boys] into two sections, taking them alternately from the list, to prevent the imputation of selection. To the first section (76) I gave belladonna; to the second (75) I gave none; the result was that two in each section were attacked by the disease. The numbers are too small to justify deductions as to the prophylactic power of belladonna, but the observation is good, because it shows how apt we are to be misled by imperfect observation. Had I given the remedy to all the boys, I should probably have attributed to it the cessation of the epidemic." (4)

Importantly, Balfour recognises the consequences of his experimental design. To divine the truth in a complex clinical setting it is essential to use a control group and that that control group be selected by chance.

This approach is, however, not immune from investigator bias. If you know which treatment the next patient is going to be allocated and you have a preference for one treatment over another then it would be simple to manipulate the clinic in order to give certain patients your favoured therapy.

All these deficiencies are largely overcome by randomisation. This process was originally employed in agricultural studies as described by Fisher (5) and was proposed for clinical trials by the eminent statistician Austin Bradford Hill in 1946 (6).

Randomisation may be unrestricted or restricted (7). Restricted randomisation methods control the probability of obtaining groups of different sizes. One example of this is the selection of treatment allocation on the basis of drawing lots or selected coloured balls from a container. The latter was used in an early trial of pre-eclampsia by Theobald in 1937 (8). In this trial 100 patients made their own treatment allocation as described in the methods section of the paper:

> "An equal number of blue and white beads were placed in a box. Each woman accepted for the experiment was asked to draw a bead from the box. Those who drew blue beads were placed in group A while those who drew white beads were placed in group B. The beads drawn out were placed in a separate container." (8)

Because the beads were not replenished, the method is a restricted form of randomisation, where the allocation to each treatment is not wholly unpredictable, and increasingly predictable, as the randomisation process proceeds.

Unrestricted or simple randomisation is the gold standard whereby each patient is assigned treatment in a completely unpredictable manner. This may be achieved most simply by the tossing of an unbiased coin or rolling of an unloaded die for each patient. However, the use of random number tables or computer programs to generate these is most frequently used in modern clinical trials. This method was most famously used in the 1948 MRC Streptomycin Trial (9, 10).

TRUE RANDOMISATION - MRC STREPTOMYCIN TRIAL

The MRC Streptomycin in Tuberculosis Trials Committee was convened in October 1946 and designed a clinical trial to evaluate the effect of bed rest plus or minus the recently discovered antibiotic streptomycin in patients with pulmonary tuberculosis. The trial, for practical reasons was not double blind or placebo controlled but patients were allocated to the two treatment arms using random sampling numbers as described in the excerpt from the paper below:

> "Determination of whether a patient would be treated by streptomycin and bed-rest (S case) or by bed-rest alone (C case) was made by reference to a statistical series based on random sampling numbers .... the details of the series were unknown to any of the investigators or to the co-ordinator and were contained in a set of sealed envelopes, each bearing on the outside only the name of the hospital and a number. After acceptance of a patient ... the appropriate numbered envelope was opened...: the card inside told if the patient was to be an S or C case, and this information was then given to the medical officer of the centre. Patients were not told before admission that they were to get special treatment; C patients did not know throughout their stay in hospital that they were control patients in a special study; they were in fact treated as they would have been in the past, the sole difference being that they had been admitted to the centre more rapidly than was normal. Usually they were not in the same wards as S patients, but the same regimen was maintained." (9)

The BMJ editorial that accompanied the publication in 1948 made a point that the randomisation used in the trial had "removed personal responsibility from the clinician" (11). What it had also done was hide from the patients' doctors what treatment they were to be allocated and indeed Chalmers points out that the real milestone represented by the MRC Streptomycin Trial was not the introduction of randomisation but this very concealment of treatment allocation (12).

The use of randomisation in clinical trials slowly spread and has now become "an essential element of trials submitted to licensing authorities for the approval of new drugs" (3). Major trials in recent years that have fundamentally changed clinical practice, such as the 1988 ISIS-2 Trial (13) that showed the benefits in patients of streptokinase and aspirin after a myocardial infarction and the 1994 4S Trial (14) that showed that statins could extend the lives of patients with coronary heart disease, have had a randomised control design. Any other methodological approach would now be almost unthinkable.

Although the MRC Streptomycin Trial was hailed by many as the first randomised controlled trial, other studies are more deserving of that honour and it is important to set this record straight. As noted by Doll (3) the MRC Whooping-cough Immunisation Trial used randomisation and commenced a few months before the Streptomycin Trial, although it was not published until three years later (15). A more serious contender is another pertussis vaccination trial conducted by the American physician Joseph Bell and reported in 1941 (16). This study involved almost a thousand children given two doses of pertussis vaccine 4 weeks apart and was begun in April 1938 in Norfolk, Virginia. As Chalmers points out, "the report of this study...is the earliest methodologically detailed account of a randomized trial..." and he goes on to quote the epidemiologist Richard Doll who described the trial as "not quite perfect, but nearly so" (17).

CONCLUSION

We can see in these examples that what we believe to be modern day innovations, and the product of inquiring and powerful intellects of the 20th century, may have their origins much earlier. This should remind us that our medical and scientific forebears were just as intelligent, just as inquiring and just as willing to put aside their prejudices and professional arrogance in a search for the truth with which to improve patient care. Van Helmont in the 17th century obviously understood the need for controlled clinical experiments and that chance must be used to determine who those controls should be. Balfour in the 19th century had a clear appreciation of how easily the clinical researcher may be misled if the data were derived from uncontrolled experiments. Theobald, Bell and Hill in the 1930s and 1940s could see that good experimental design must include randomisation of subjects to active treatment and control arms in order to ensure a fair evaluation of the therapy in question. Without controls and without allowing chance to determine which patient received which treatment the study would yield potentially meaningless and perhaps even clinically dangerous results.

Van Helmont began this process of methodological development in clinical trials with a simple wager. True randomisation in clinical trials did have to wait until the 20th century to be implemented, but whether it was through the use of coloured beads, the roll of dice, the tossing of a coin or the use of random numbers we can now be confident that the results of a well conducted randomised controlled trial will provide us with the best standard of evidence we can hope for to guide clinical practice.

REFERENCES

1. Van Helmont JB. *Oriatrike, or physick refined: the common errors therein refuted and the whole are reformed and rectified.* London: Lodowick-Loyd, 1662: 526.

2. Amberson JB, McMahon BT, Pinner M. A clinical trial of sanocrysin in pulmonary tuberculosis. *American Review of Tuberculosis* 1931; 24: 401-35.

3. Doll R. Controlled trials: the 1948 watershed. *British Medical Journal* 1998; 317: 1217-20.

4. Balfour TG. Quoted in West C (1854). Lectures on the Diseases of Infancy and Childhood. London, Longman, Brown, Green and Longmans, p 600. http://www.jameslindlibrary.org/trial_records/19t h_Century/balfour/balfour_kp.html (Accessed May 9, 2009).

5. Fisher RA. The arrangement of field experiments. *Journal of the Ministry of Agriculture* 1926; 33: 503-13.

6. Hill AB. Memories of the British streptomycin trial in tuberculosis. *Controlled Clinical Trials* 1990; 11: 77-9.

7. Grimes DA, Schulz KF. Generation of allocation sequences in randomised controlled trials: chance not choice. *Lancet* 2002; 359: 515-9.

8. Theobald GW. Effect of calcium and vitamin A and D on incidence of pregnancy toxaemia. *Lancet* 1937; 2: 1397-9.

9. Medical Research Council. Streptomycin treatment of pulmonary tuberculosis: a Medical Research Council investigation. *British Medical Journal* 1948; 2: 769-82.
    http://bmj.com/content/vol317/issue7167

10. Yoshioka A. Use of randomisation in the Medical Research Council's clinical trial of streptomycin in

pulmonary tuberculosis in the 1940s. *British Medical Journal* 1998; 317: 1220-3.

11. Editorial. The controlled therapeutic trial. *British Medical Journal* 1948; 2: 791-2.

12. Chalmers I. Comparing like with like: some historical milestones in the evolution of methods to create unbiased comparison groups in therapeutic experiments. *International Journal of Epidemiology* 2001; 30: 1170-8.

13. ISIS-2 Collaborative Group. Randomised trial of intravenous streptokinase, oral aspirin, both, or neither among 17187 cases of suspected acute myocardial infarction: ISIS-2. *Lancet* 1988; 2: 349-360.

14. 4S Group. Randomised trial of cholesterol lowering in 4444 patients with coronary heart disease: the Scandinavian Simvastatin Survival Study (4S) *Lancet* 1994; 344:1383-9.

15. Medical Research Council. The prevention of whooping-cough by vaccination. BMJ 1951,1:1463-71.

16. Bell JA. Pertussis prophylaxis with two doses of alum-precipitated vaccine. *Public Health Reports* 1941; 56: 1535-46.

17. Chalmers I. Joseph Asbury Bell and the birth of randomized trials. 2006 The James Lind Library www.jameslindlibrary.org (Accessed May 9, 2009)

4

FRANKLIN AND MAGNETISM:

the importance of blinding and placebos in clinical trials

In pre-revolutionary France, the unwell who were also well-to-do had an interesting and novel therapeutic option. In 1778 a charismatic German physician called Franz Anton Mesmer had arrived in Paris from Vienna and his medical reputation had preceded him (fig.5).

What sort of treatment did this new doctor offer and what could you expect at his hands? Although the therapy he and his followers offered was shrouded in mystery there are several contemporary accounts and from these we may reconstruct as session with Mesmer (1,2).

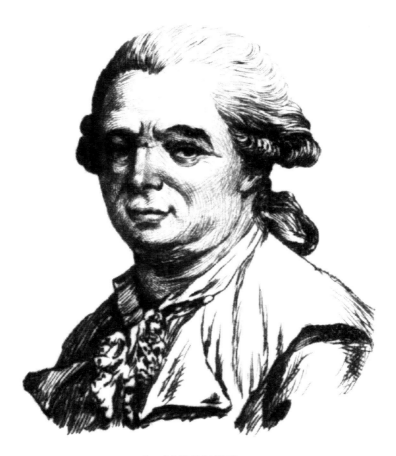

A MESMER

Figure 5. Portrait of Franz Anton Mesmer (1734-1815).

His 'clinic' was in the exclusive Place Vendôme in Paris – a square in the 1st arrondissement and now home to the Ritz Hotel. There you would enter a dimly lit room and join as many as thirty other patients seated in concentric circles. In the centre of the room was a *baquet*, an oval wooden tub approximately 120 cm long and 30 cm deep. This was filled with a mixture of ground glass and iron fillings and contained bottles of water that had been 'magnetized'. The tub had a wooden lid with a series of holes through which were passed angled metal rods. Each patient would hold one of these rods and could place it on their affected body part. Your fellow patients would be suffering from a range of ills for Mesmer advocated his treatment for the cure of all afflictions except venereal diseases. In the background there would be hushed silence punctuated by the ethereal sounds from the glass armonica – a newly invented musical instrument that sounded like a wet finger stroking the rim of a wine glass.

When the scene was set, Mesmer himself would appear in a lilac silk coat carrying a metal wand. As he circled the room he would select patients with whom he sat *en rapport* – directly in front of them, toes and knees touching and gazing intently into their eyes. His assistants, who are reported to have been young and handsome, would also help the 'magnetic flux' by massaging patients between their knees, on their backs and lightly on their breasts. The combination of these sensory stimuli caused many patients to become entranced or 'mesmerised' and some to faint or convulse. And, of course, many claimed to be cured.

But what was really happening here? Lighting, music, costume, drama and sensuality – what was going on was more ritual than medicine, more suggestion than treatment, more Dumbledore than doctoring. Perhaps in a pre-enlightenment era, this would simply have been viewed as magic. But, this was the 1780s – the world had moved on. Descartes had taught us to be rationalists,

Newton had explained the invisible forces that controlled the universe, and Voltaire, who had only recently died had, with his customary wit, urged us to be altogether more sensible. Now, this 'magic' had to have a rational scientific basis and Mesmer provided it. It is quite clear what Mesmer himself believed was happening. During his time in Vienna he had experimented with the use of conventional magnetic therapy, using steel magnets to treat patients. However, he had moved beyond this and abandoned the use of metal devices in favour of channeling and realigning the 'animal' rather than 'mineral' magnetism he believed to be inherent in us all. He believed that magnetic fluid flowed from the stars into all living things and that all disease was the result of an obstruction to this flow. His task as a physician was to correct these obstructions, which he believed he could do without the use of conventional magnets. Mesmer's explanation is now widely discredited and most modern historians believe that he was in fact hypnotizing his patients and was also making use of powerful placebo effects.

Despite the facts that we now believe Mesmer and his associates were inducing a trance-like state in their patients, and even that we now use mesmerism as a synonym for hypnotism, Mesmer himself never claimed to be a hypnotist. He was adamant that there was a rationale and physical explanation for the cures he claimed to effect (3).

Mesmer and his followers including Deslon, the French physician to the brother of Louis XVI, soon became the height of fashion, but his treatment was not without its critics. Mesmer was anxious to gain acceptance by the medical and scientific establishment in Paris, some say to vindicate his beliefs, others to ensure his income. But, the establishment in the form of the Society of Medicine would have nothing to do with him (1).

22222

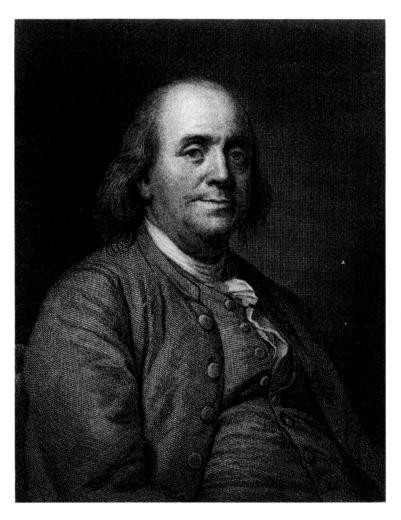

Figure 6.   Benjamin Franklin (1706-1790). Engraving: H. B. Hall from the original picture in Passel painted from life by J.A. Duplessis in 1783.

Interestingly, although we may regard Mesmer as a quack today, his approach was not completely without merit in the field of clinical trials. In 1780, in an attempt to persuade the above Society of the worth of his technique, he proposed a trial of a remarkably modern design (4). Twenty-four patients would be randomly assigned to either orthodox medicine or mesmerism and the results would be adjudicated by an independent panel. His proposal was, however, ignored.

ROYAL COMMISSION

Instead, the King himself stepped in and appointed commissions to investigate and report on Mesmer's claims. Thus, an elderly American statesman in the form of the Ambassador to France, Benjamin Franklin, enters the story (fig. 6). In truth he had already met Mesmer, having dined with him in 1779 (1) and had heard much about him and his practices. Franklin was a scientist, among many other things, and had a scientist's scepticism. When asked by a sick friend in 1784 whether he should consult Mesmer, Franklin wrote:

> "…there being so many Disorders which cure themselves, and such a Disposition in Mankind to deceive themselves and one another on these Occasions; and this living long having given me frequent Opportunities of seeing certain Remedies cry'd up as curing every thing, and yet soon after totally laid aside as useless, I cannot but fear that the Expectations of great Advantage from this new Method of treating Diseases, will prove a Delusion." (5)

Here we have an appreciation that self-delusion may be at the root of the "new method". Interestingly, however, this was not the first time that Franklin had written presciently about the placebo effect. Almost three decades earlier, in 1757, as part of his investigations into the therapeutic effects of electricity,

Franklin had conducted experiments giving electric shocks to patients suffering from paralysis. Some of Franklin's patients seemed to benefit, at least in the short term, but his scepticism forbade him from drawing a clear line of causality from the treatment to its effect. He knew that the maxim *post hoc ergo propter hoc* was not necessarily true. He speculated on the possible causes of the observed benefits when he wrote to John Pringle and the Royal Society:

> "...I never knew any Advantage from Electricity in Palsies that was permanent. And how far the apparent temporary Advantage might arise from the Exercise in the Patients Journey and coming daily to my House, or from the Spirits given by the Hope of Success, enabling them to exert more Strength in moving their Limbs, I will not pretend to say."
> (6)

Here again, as in his letter of 1784, we have the appreciation that what we would call today the placebo effect may have accounted for the observed benefits.

And it was this that the Royal Commission set out to investigate. They did not, however, examine Mesmer's technique directly – he refused to be studied. Instead they focused on an evaluation of the scientific basis for his claims. Mesmer professed to be an instrument to channel and realign the natural magnetic fluxes. If the existence, or awareness, of such fluxes could be disproved then Mesmer's approach could be dismissed as groundless.

The commission's approach is outlined in their report which was published in 1784 (7) and a modern English translation is available (8). Franklin and his colleagues devised a series of experiments using a blinded design for the first time. Subjects (including the commissioners themselves) were blindfolded and presented with 'magnetised' or 'mesmerised' objects and with objects that had not been manipulated in such a way. The subjects were unable to distinguish the two and variably reported the effects – usually reporting the effects of mesmerism only when told that this was happening, whether or not it in fact was. Bailly reports:

> "We succeeded in manipulating the imagination. Without being touched or signaled, the subjects who thought themselves magnetized felt pain, felt heat, a very great heat. In some cases we provoked convulsions and what is known as crises." (quoted in 1)

The commission also employed placebos in the form of 'mesmerised' water and even 'mesmerised' trees. The latter being used to see if subjects could indeed identify a normal tree from one that had been magnetised. They could not.

As a result of these blinded and placebo controlled experiments the commission was able to conclude that there was no basis to Mesmer's claims – they could not demonstrate the existence or awareness in subjects of animal magnetism. Instead they explained that 'animal magnetism' "owed its apparent efficacy to the power of suggestion in susceptible or naïve individuals." (2)

PLACEBOS

Although the term placebo did not enter medical parlance until 1785 when it was included in a medical dictionary for the first time (9) it is clear that for centuries, if not millennia, before, healers had used remedies that they knew to have no active ingredients, but which they also knew would appease their patients. Placebo indeed is Latin for, 'I shall please'. However, Franklin and the French Royal Commissioners are credited with being the first to use placebos in a clinical research setting.

Soon after their studies in 1784 another involving a placebo-controlled strategy was designed by the English physician John Haygarth (10). He was interested in the claims made by the American physician Elisha Perkins regarding the use of metal devices called Tractors. These devices were made from secret alloys and similar in appearance to spatulae. Perkins claimed that applying these to patients could cure various ills. Haygarth was skeptical and proposed the following test:

> "Let [the Tractors'] merit be impartially investigated, in order to support their fame, if it be well-founded, or to correct the public opinion, if merely formed upon delusion…..Prepare a pair of false, exactly to resemble the true Tractors. Let the secret be kept inviolable, not only from the patient but also from any other person. Let the efficacy of both be impartially tried and the reports of the effects produced by the true and false Tractors be fully given in the words of the patients." (quoted in 10)

The proposed single-blind placebo controlled study was carried out by Haygarth's colleagues in Bath and the genuine and sham Tractors were found to be equally effective, or indeed ineffective. Haygarth concluded in his pamphlet of 1800, "Imagination can cause, as well as cure, diseases of the body" (11).

Both Franklin and Haygarth were interested in evaluating devices, but placebos have been even more widely used in the evaluation of pharmacological preparations. Possibly the earliest trial to use a placebo-controlled design comparing an 'active' treatment with an 'inactive' placebo was that conducted in 1835 by the well-named Society of Truth Loving Men (12). They set out to test the claims of homeopaths in the city of Nuremberg and prepared a set of vials − half containing water, and half a diluted salt solution. The vials were shuffled and given to 47 volunteers who had been informed of the nature and design of the experiment. They were asked to take the liquid in their allotted vial and report back any unusual effects. The results failed to confirm any therapeutic effects of the 'active' treatment and the investigators concluded that the claims of the homeopaths "were the fruit of imagination, self-deception and preconceived opinion – if not fraud." (13)

Placebos are now an essential part of modern clinical research, both to mask the treatment allocation and to prevent confounding from the so-called placebo effect, i.e. the effects that an inactive substance, procedure or device may have when administered in a clinical context over and above the effects observed of no treatment.

The placebo effect is complex and still relatively poorly understood (9), but it is undoubtedly real and can have significant impact on the evaluations of different medical treatments if it is not taken into account. Whatever the treatment – medication, medical device, surgery or psychological intervention – it may be possible to create a matched but ineffective alternative. Benefit may usually only be claimed if the active treatment produces significantly greater benefit than the placebo. Of course it is not always ethical to use a placebo. If there is an established therapy for any given disease it would be quite unethical to withhold that treatment and administer a placebo in its place. In these circumstances it is necessary to compare one active treatment with another in a head-to-head fashion. While placebo-controlled studies are highly regarded they are not the only source of robust clinical data, a fact acknowledged even by regulatory and licensing authorities in the evaluation of new drugs for example.

BLINDING

The use of placebo controls and blinding of treatment allocation are inextricably linked in modern clinical research. Franklin and his colleagues literally blindfolded their subjects to prevent them seeing whether they were being 'magnetised' or not, while Haygarth proposed the construction of matched placebo devices in the form of the sham Tractors in order to 'blind' the patients to their treatment. In both these examples the investigators knew what was going on while the patients did not. Such a single-blind approach is still widely used, but where practicable a double-blind is preferred. In such cases neither investigator nor subject is aware of the treatment allocation and thus the potential for bias introduced by the investigator is eliminated. Kaptchuk appropriately refers to this as 'shared ignorance' (14) and while it is often a difficult concept to explain to potential recruits into a clinical trial, it has become the cornerstone of the modern randomised controlled clinical trial and is regarded as the gold-standard for the acquisition of meaningful and scientifically robust clinical data.

In the use of both single and double-blind experimental designs there is a necessity for deception. This could never be acceptable as part of routine medical care, but in the very different environment of a clinical trial such an approach is not only acceptable but legitimate and desirable. There is of course one important caveat to this and that is that the patient should be fully informed of the study design, the use of placebos and the use of blinding before taking part in the study. If the patient consents at the outset to such a 'deception' then the ethical concerns largely evaporate. However, the 'moral discomfort' experienced by clinician-scientists in this setting may need to be addressed (15). This may be a problem particularly in studies with a single-blind design and especially those involving sham procedures to be performed. The discomfort arises because the clinician who is normally responsible for patient care in a setting that is free from subterfuge suddenly finds herself in one where she is expected to act a part and merely pretend to treat her patient. If the study design is double blind, these feelings are largely alleviated for the clinician because in this case she is just as ignorant of the treatment being administered as the subject.

IMPORTANCE TODAY

The double-blind, placebo controlled randomised clinical trial is regarded by many as one of the single greatest achievements in medicine. Without such a powerful tool our clinical practice may be based on observation and experience, but not on hard irrefutable evidence. Although we had to wait until the 20th century for the first rigorous double-blind, placebo controlled randomised clinical trials, the story – at least concerning the notions of blinding and placebo control – began, as we have seen, two centuries before. Advances in medicine, although routinely portrayed as overnight occurrences in the media, are often the products of a painfully slow gestation. Medicine, today, would simply not be what it is if it were not for the use of trial designs that eliminate, as far as possible, bias introduced by both the patient and the investigator. Without the ingenuity of a group of enlightened French scientists led by an aging American diplomat perhaps we would not have been able to enjoy the fruits of such trials. And, perhaps physicians would still have wands.

REFERENCES

1. Lopez C-A. Franklin and Mesmer: an encounter. *Yale Journal of Biology and Medicine* 1993; 66: 325-31.

2. Macklis RM. Magnetic healing, quackery, and the debate about the health effects of electromagnetic fields. *Annals of Internal Medicine* 1993; 118: 376-83.

3. Mesmer FA. Magnétisme animal. Mémoires et aphorismes de Mesmer, Adamant Media Corporation, 2002.

4. Donaldson IML. Mesmer's 1780 proposal for a controlled trial to test his method of treatment using 'animal magnetism'. *Journal of the Royal Society of Medicine* 2005; 98: 572-5.

5. Letter from Franklin to la Sublière de la Condamine, March 19, 1784. Franklin Collection, Yale University. http://franklinpapers.org/franklin/framedVolumes.jsp (Accessed May 20, 2009)

6. Letter from Franklin to John Pringle, December 21, 1757. Franklin Collection, Yale University. http://franklinpapers.org/franklin/framedNames.jsp (Accessed May 21, 2009)

7. Rapport des commissionaires chargé par le Roi, de l'examen du magnétisme animale. Imprimé par ordre du Roi. [Report of the commissioners charged by the King with the examination of animal magnetism. Printed by order of the King] Paris : L'Imprimerie Royale, 1784.

8. Franklin B, Majault, Le Roy, Sallin, Bailly JS, D'Arcet, de Bory, Guillotin JI, Lavoisier A. Report of the commissioners charged by the King with the examination of animal magnetism. 1784. *International Journal of Clinical and Experimental Hypnosis* 2002; 50: 332-63.

9. de Craen AJM, Kaptchuk TJ, Tijssen JGP, Kleijnen J. Placebos and placebo effects in medicine: historical overview. *Journal of the Royal Society of Medicine* 1999; 92: 511-5.

10. Booth CC. John Haygarth FRS (1740-1827). The James Lind Library 2002 www.jameslindlibrary.org (Accessed May 21, 2009)

11. Haygarth J. Of the imagination, as a cause and as a cure of disorders of the body: exemplified by fictitious tractors, and epidemical convulsions. Bath: R. Crutwell, 1800.

12. Stolberg M. Inventing the randomized double-blind trial: The Nuremberg salt test of 1835. The James Lind Library 2006 www.jameslindlibrary.org (Accessed May 21, 2009)

13. Löhner G, on behalf of a society of truth-loving men. Die homöopathischen Kochsalzversuche zu Nürnberg [The homeopathic salt trials in Nuremberg]. Nuremberg, 1835.

14. Kaptchuk TJ. Intentional ignorance: a history of blind assessment and placebo controls in medicine. *Bulletin of the History of Medicine* 1998; 72: 389-433.

15. Miller FG, Kaptchuk TJ. Sham procedures and the ethics of clinical trials. *Journal of the Royal Society of Medicine* 2004; 97: 576-8.

5

CLINTON AND THE APOLOGY:

the importance of trust in clinical trials

In 1997 President Bill Clinton stood in the East Room of the White House and apologised (1). The misdemeanour was not some indiscretion committed by the incumbent of the Oval Office, but rather a much more important and far reaching crime that began a lifetime before in Tuskegee, Alabama.

THE TUSKEGEE SYPHILIS STUDY

If you were to drive through the city of Tuskegee today you would see a small, relatively poor, University town with African-Americans making up more than 95% of the population (2). In 1932, during the depression, it was chosen as the centre of an observational study conducted by the US Public Health Service into the sexually transmitted disease, syphilis (3). This government body set up a health screening programme performing blood tests and asking questions that quickly recruited around 400 poor, black, and mostly illiterate farm workers who all tested positive for syphilis. For participating in the study, the men were told they would be given free medical examinations, free hot meals and free burial insurance.

Now, there is immediate controversy as to whether the participants in this study were aware of what was going on, and what it was exactly they had signed up for (3-5). The term syphilis was never mentioned; rather the term "bad blood" was used (5). This may have been a well understood euphemism for the venereal disease, which was, at the time, incurable. Alternatively, it may have been a deception employed by the investigators. The truth of the matter is debatable, but what is not a matter of discussion is the intent of the investigators and the complete abuse of trust they perpetrated on the study participants (6). When these farm workers were told they were suffering from "bad blood" they were also told that they needed treatment, but the investigators lied when they said they would provide it as part of the study.

This "treatment" would in reality consist of regular tests – some highly invasive such as lumbar punctures – and would not constitute therapy of any kind (fig. 7). Some men were given drug therapy, but at doses so low as to ensure that no effect would be seen. When the study was begun there was no effective treatment for syphilis. However, when penicillin became available in the 1940s, the study subjects were effectively denied this treatment because it was not in the interests of the investigators to tell them they had syphilis or to provide a potential cure. Antibiotics may not have helped the later stages of syphilis that many of the men developed, but they may have

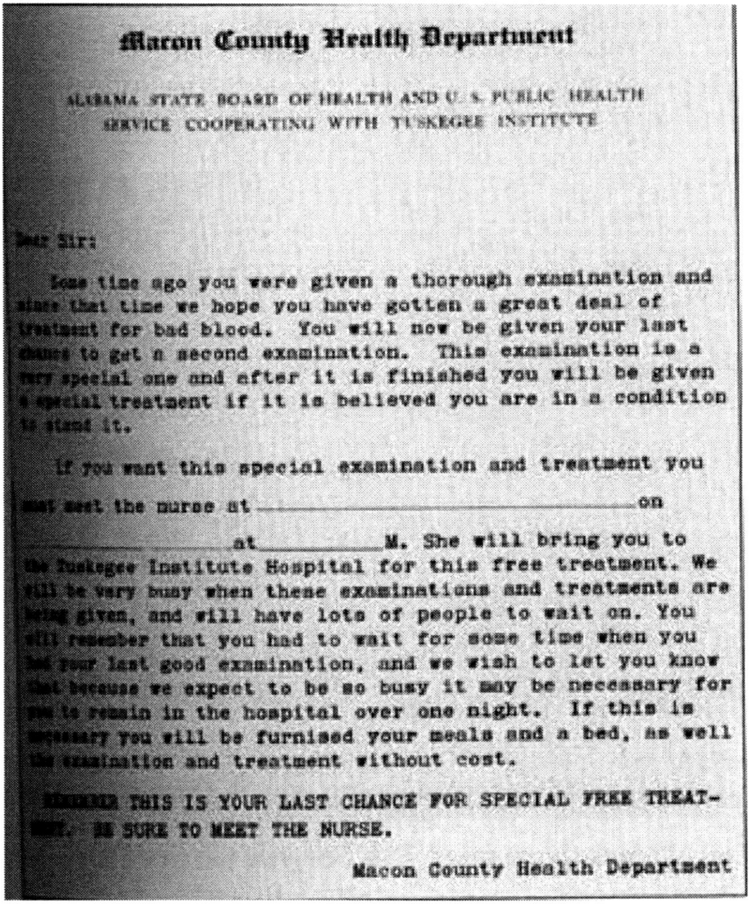

Macon County Health Department

ALABAMA STATE BOARD OF HEALTH AND U. S. PUBLIC HEALTH
SERVICE COOPERATING WITH TUSKEGEE INSTITUTE

Dear Sir:

Some time ago you were given a thorough examination and
since that time we hope you have gotten a great deal of
treatment for bad blood. You will now be given your last
chance to get a second examination. This examination is a
very special one and after it is finished you will be given
a special treatment if it is believed you are in a condition
to stand it.

If you want this special examination and treatment you
must meet the nurse at _____ on
_____ at _____ M. She will bring you to
the Tuskegee Institute Hospital for this free treatment. We
will be very busy when these examinations and treatments are
being given, and will have lots of people to wait on. You
will remember that you had to wait for some time when you
had your last good examination, and we wish to let you know
that because we expect to be so busy it may be necessary for
you to remain in the hospital over one night. If this is
necessary you will be furnised your meals and a bed, as well
the examination and treatment without cost.

REMEMBER THIS IS YOUR LAST CHANCE FOR SPECIAL FREE TREAT-
MENT. BE SURE TO MEET THE NURSE.

                                    Macon County Health Department

Figure 7.   Copy of letter sent to Tuskegee Syphilis Study
participants inviting them to a "special examination and treatment".
Lumbar punctures were performed on those who attended. (US
Government material)

prevented the spread of the disease to others in the community. Wives, partners and children, newly infected by the Tuskegee men, were not offered treatment because studying the spread of the disease was one of the objectives of the investigators. Apart from the denial of drug therapy, no form of counselling was given to the men to avoid the spread of syphilis to their families because the fact that they had the disease was never mentioned.

In fact it was the length to which the investigators went to prevent their subjects being treated that has been amongst the most damning criticisms of the study (6). For example, at the outbreak of war a number of the Tuskegee men registered for military service. They were tested for syphilis as part of their military induction, found to be positive and ordered to receive penicillin. When the US Public Health Service discovered this they arranged for the men to be exempted from service, thus ensuring that no treatment was given (5,6). Why did they go to these lengths? Simply because the purpose of this study was not, after all, to investigate treatments for syphilis in humans, it was to investigate the natural history of the disease in the black population, how it spread, and, in short, to see how these men would die.

At the time one of the Tuskegee Study investigators stated, "As I see it we have no further interest in these patients until they die" (5,6) What was implicit was the interest of the investigators in receiving the autopsy reports of all study subjects.

THE END OF THE STUDY

The study went on for 40 years, and did not come to an end because of some corporate awakening within the US Public Health Service as to the immorality of the study, but because it was exposed in the media. Peter Buxton, a venereal disease interviewer and investigator for the US Public Health Service, who had been attempting to raise the issue within his organisation since 1966, blew the whistle and spoke to the press. (5) On July 26, 1972 the New York Times led with the headline: "Syphilis Victims in U.S. Study Went Untreated for 40 Years", and the accompanying front page story detailed, "the longest non-therapeutic experiment on human beings in medical history". (4)

By this time, 28 of the men had died directly of syphilis, 100 were dead of related complications, 40 of their wives had been infected, and 19 of their children had been born with congenital syphilis. (6) A year later, the National Association for the Advancement of Colored People (NAACP) filed a class-action lawsuit and won a US$10 million out of court settlement that was divided among the study's participants. In addition, free health care was given to the surviving men, and to the infected wives, widows and children.

With regard to the Tuskegee Syphilis experiment, the Los Angeles Times later noted that the US Public Health Service had persuaded hundreds of black men to become "human guinea pigs", and then qualified that statement by saying:

> "Well, perhaps not quite that, because the doctors obviously did not regard their subjects as completely human." (7)

This speculation proved to be correct, for when, in 1976, the historian James Jones interviewed John Heller, Director of the Venereal Diseases Unit of the US Public Health Service from 1943 to 1948, Heller remarked: "The [Tuskegee] men's status did not warrant ethical debate. They were subjects, not patients; clinical material, not sick people" (5).

This encapsulates the lesson to be learned from the Tuskegee Study. Sometimes and for some reasons investigators forget that the subjects they are studying are human, with all the rights and claims to dignity that this entails. When investigators forget this most basic tenet, things go terribly wrong and the potential for atrocity becomes a reality (8).

It is more than reasonable to expect the physician investigator, who has after all sworn the Hippocratic Oath, to abide by the highest professional standards and behave at all times in an ethical manner. However, the evidence appears to the contrary, and the echo of Tuskegee should ring in our ears and remind us that this is not enough. Patients and trial subjects need more protection than this.

When we remember Tuskegee we are not revisiting the distant past. This all happened only 40 years ago in the most sophisticated healthcare system on the globe, where a group of underprivileged and vulnerable men and their families were simply exploited in the dubious attempt to advance science. This was not acceptable then, and it is certainly not now. The multi-layers of internationally agreed guidelines and nationally enforced legislation have reiterated this again and again. The Declaration of Helsinki, a document primarily drafted to guide physicians, has stated since 1964, "The health of my patient will be my first consideration" (9), and the ICH-GCP guidelines go even further:

> "The rights, safety, and well-being of the trial subjects are the most important considerations and should prevail over the interests of science and society." (10)

The late Thomas Clark Chalmers, an early advocate of the importance of randomised controlled clinical trials and the usefulness of meta-analyses, put it simply and practically:

"I think the major ethical principle is that you shouldn't be involved in a trial unless you would be willing to be randomized yourself if you had the disease." (11)

It is hard to imagine that Tuskegee could have happened if the US Public Health Service investigators had adhered to this maxim when designing and conducting their Study.

THE LEGACY OF TUSKEGEE

The legacy of Tuskegee has been debated. The extent of its impact on the conduct and oversight of clinical trials in the US is undeniable. Tuskegee has been described as America's Nuremberg (12) and the overhaul of legislation that took place in its wake to ensure that it could not happen again was long overdue. Most tangibly was the 1974 creation of the National Commission for the Protection of Human Subjects in Biomedical and Behavioral Research and the National Research Act. This act required all institutions in receipt of federal funding to establish Institutional Review Boards or ethical committees (13) However, more insidiously, the adverse legacy of Tuskegee may be found in the deep mistrust that African-Americans have for medical authority in the US and the persistent failure of attempts to increase the representation of ethnic minorities in clinical research (13).

Since its discovery, the Tuskegee Syphilis Experiment has seldom been out of the press, but in February 1997 the story was given a new audience when a television adaptation of the play *Miss Ever's Boys* by David Feldshuh was broadcast on the cable network HBO in the US. This programme was watched by an estimated 3 million African-American households (14). Perhaps the focus given to the story by this dramatisation and the ensuing discussion prompted the authorities to take the action with which we began this chapter. Clinton's public apology just three months later can be viewed sceptically, but it was undoubtedly needed if any healing was to take place.

President Clinton delivered the apology in person to the last five surviving Tuskegee men who were present at the White House and to three others by satellite, who were too frail to travel from Alabama. He said that what the government had done was deeply, profoundly and morally wrong.

He went on:

> "To the survivors, to the wives and family members, the children and the grandchildren, I say what you know: No power on Earth can give you back the lives lost, the pain suffered, the years of internal torment and anguish.
>
> What was done cannot be undone. But we can end the silence. We can stop turning our heads away. We can look at you in the eye and finally say, on behalf of the American people: what the United States government did was shameful.
>
> And I am sorry." (1)

CONCLUSION

Ethics in clinical trials are about many things, but first and foremost they are about remembering that the participants of our studies are people just like us. They are not "clinical material" or laboratory animals, they are human beings. At the core of the Tuskegee scandal was a basic disregard and lack of respect for the equality and humanity of mankind. Without such respect anything becomes possible in the name of medical science. Firmly applying the basic ethical principles now codified in law (15), will help ensure these possibilities are rendered impossible, and that the past cannot happen again.

REFERENCES

1. Remarks by the President in apology for study done in Tuskegee. The White House. Office of the Press Secretary May 16, 1997. http://www.cdc.gov/nchstp/od/tuskegee/clinton p.htm (Accessed June 17, 2009).
2. http://www.elook.org/city/cities/Tuskegee_Alaba ma.html (Accessed June 17, 2009).
3. US Public Health Service. Final report of the Tuskegee Syphilis Study Ad Hoc Advisory Panel. Washington DC: US Dept of Health, Education, and Welfare, Public Health Service, 1973.
4. Heller J. Syphilis victims in U.S. study went untreated for 40 years. *New York Times* July 26, 1972.
5. Jones, J. *Bad blood: The Tuskegee syphilis experiment: A tragedy of race and medicine.* NY: The Free Press, 1981.
6. Brunner B. The Tuskegee Syphilis Experiment. Tuskegee University http://www.tuskegee.edu/ Global/Story.asp?s=1207586 (Accessed June 17, 2009).
7. Brown, P. Perspectives in Medical Sociology 2nd Edition. Waveland Press, Prospect Heights, 1996.
8. Gaw A. Beyond consent: the potential for atrocity. *Journal of the Royal Society of Medicine* 2006; 99: 175-7.
9. Declaration of Helsinki. http://www.wma.net/e/policy/b3.htm (Accessed June 17, 2009).

10. ICH-GCP[2.3]
    http://www.ich.org/LOB/media/MEDIA482.pdf
    (Accessed June 17, 2009)
11. Spencer S. Thomas C. Chalmers: faculty profile.
    Healthy News. 1984; 4:2.
12. Wolinsky H. Steps still being taken to undo damage
    of "America's Nuremberg". *Annals of Internal
    Medicine* 1997; 127: I43-4.
13. Corbie-Smith G. The continuing legacy of the
    Tuskegee Syphilis Study: considerations for clinical
    investigation. *American Journal of Medical Science*
    1999; 317: 5-8.
14. Sargent J. (Director) *Miss Evers' Boys*, HBO Debut.
    Home Box Office, 1997.
15. Statutory Instrument 2004 No. 1031. The
    Medicines for Human Use (Clinical Trials)
    Regulations 2004. http://www.hmso.gov.uk/si/
    si2004/20041031.htm (Accessed June 17, 2009)

6

TAYLOR AND THE NAZIS:

the importance of codes of practice in clinical trials

It was with disbelief that the post-war world received news of medical experiments performed on the inmates of concentration camps in Nazi Germany (1). The subsequent trial in Nuremberg of 23 defendants, 20 of whom were medically qualified, yielded 16 guilty verdicts and 7 death sentences. In his opening remarks at the trial in Nuremberg Brigadier General Telford Taylor (fig. 8), the American Chief of Council, noted:

> 'To kill, to maim, and to torture is criminal under all modern systems of law . . . yet these [physician] defendants, all of whom were fully able to comprehend the nature of their acts . . . are responsible for wholesale murder and unspeakably cruel tortures.' (2)

During the eight-month trial a detailed catalogue of medical experimentation was presented to the court (2, 3). For example, in Dachau between 1942–1944 there was a series of experiments designed to examine aspects of aviation medicine, involving high-altitude experiments, the effects of freezing water baths and the enforced drinking of seawater. In Buchenwald and Ravensbrück throughout the war, a series of studies examined the simulation and treatment of battlefield injuries, such as exposure to mustard gas, phosphorus burns, bone transplantation, and sulfanilimide treatments. In Dachau, Buchenwald and Sachsenhausen during 1941–1945 there were a variety of infectious disease studies involving the deliberate infection of inmates with malaria, epidemic jaundice and typhus. Finally, in Auschwitz, Buchenwald and Ravensbrück there were a number of eugenic and lethal experiments involving sterilization and poisoned bullets.

The trial, *United States of America v. Karl Brandt et al* – more commonly known as the Doctors' Trial – began on 9th December 1946 (4). Brandt (fig. 9) was the most senior defendant, having been Hitler's personal physician since 1934 and appointed by him in 1942 as Plenipotentiary for Health and Medical Services and in 1943 as General Commissioner for Sanitation and Health, thus explicitly extending his authority to the field of medical science and research (2).

The 23 German physicians and administrators tried at Nuremberg were indicted on four counts:

1. conspiracy to commit war crimes and crimes against humanity
2. war crimes (i.e., crimes against persons protected by the laws of war, such as prisoners of war)
3. crimes against humanity (including persons not protected by the laws of war)

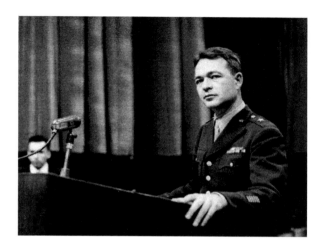

Figure 8. Brigadier General Telford Taylor, Doctors' Trial Nuremberg 1947.

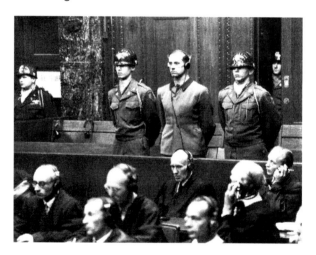

Figure 9. Dr Karl Brandt in the dock at the Doctors' Trial, Nuremberg 1947.

4. membership of a criminal organization (the SS) (4).

The defendants were charged with ordering, supervising, or coordinating criminal activities, as well as participating in them directly (4).

THE NUREMBERG CODE

On August 19th, 1947, the Nuremberg judges delivered their verdict to the defendants. As a preamble to this judgement they realised the need to address the question of medical experiments involving human beings in more general terms. This statement contained ten principles detailing common research practices when humans are involved and was set out in a section of their judgement entitled: 'Permissable Medical Experiments' (5). Pivotal to the ethical approach advocated in this statement was the need to obtain informed consent before any research procedure was carried out. These ten standards later became known as the Nuremberg Code and as Shuster noted: "[it] combined Hippocratic ethics and the protection of human rights" (6). The Nuremberg code is widely regarded as the predecessor to all modern codes of ethical practice in clinical research that followed, and the first to be internationally recognized.

But who devised this set of standards? There is some confusion as to the author, or authors, of the code (7). As noted above, it was presented by the judges presiding over the Doctors' Trial, but American military physicians, Leo Alexander and Andrew Ivy, made significant contributions.

Two days before the start of the trial Leo Alexander, a prominent American neurologist who was the chief medical advisor, sent a memorandum to Telford Taylor. This memorandum entitled "Ethical and non-ethical experimentation on human beings" detailed three main principles which should be taken into account when carrying out experiments involving humans. The first of these principles focussed on the notion of a valid and informed consent by a willing volunteer. The second of these principles revisited the duty of physicians expressed in the Hippocratic Oath. Alexander stated: "the medical Hippocratic attitude prohibits an experiment if the foregone conclusion, probability or *a priori* reason to believe exists, that death or disabling injury of the experimental subject will occur." The third of these principles entailed the ensuring of good clinical practices. These included a sound experimental design and for the experiment to be carried out by groups of competent researchers. Alexander also suggested that the experiment should be based on previous experiments carried out on non-human subjects, i.e. animals. In this way the researchers would know roughly the expected results and take measures to minimise the harm to any subjects.

Several months later, on April 15th 1947, a second memorandum followed. In this memo he outlined what he felt were the six basic rules for conducting medical experiments in an ethical manner. These included "valid voluntary consent on the part of the subject, with there being an absence of duress and sufficient disclosure on the part of the experimenter regarding the nature and possible consequences of the experiment" (7).

It is clear from examination of the two memoranda sent by Alexander to Taylor that Alexander's role in the development of the code was instrumental. Alexander highlighted the need for a code of some description detailing many of the practices which should be taken into consideration when conducting medical experiments on human beings. If we compare the memoranda written by Alexander with the Nuremberg Code itself, it is equally clear that all of the concepts contained in Alexander's notes can be found in the Nuremberg Code with even much of the language used by him adopted in the Code.

Andrew Ivy was a well-known physiologist who was asked to be medical adviser to the prosecution at the trial of the United States of America vs. Karl Brandt et al (8). Ivy was a suitable choice because he had a good knowledge of the experiments conducted on American prisoners in the Stateville Prison in Illinois, his home state, which the Nazi doctors claimed were conducted in the same manner to the experiments they carried out on concentration camp prisoners. In Ivy's testimony to the court he put forward three key principles which he had devised on behalf of the American Medical Association. These key principles were contained in a document entitled "Principles of Ethics Concerning Experimentation with Human Beings". He believed that these three principles were shared by all in the medical profession and should become common practice in the conduct of experiments when humans are involved.

In summary Ivy's three principles were:

1. the need for free, informed consent

2. the scientifically robust design of experiments based on results of animal experimentation and on a knowledge of the natural history of the disease under study

3. the conduct of experiments only by scientifically qualified persons

Comparisons can be drawn and obvious similarities noted between the principles put forward by Ivy and those contained in the memoranda sent to Taylor by Alexander. The judges at Nuremberg clearly took note of the counsel they received from both men and their contributions provided the foundations of the Nuremberg code (2,7).

POST WAR EXPERIMENTATION

Even with the development of a formal code of practice, adherence to the Nuremberg Code was not automatically assured. Many in the medical profession, while seeing the code as appropriate to Nazi doctors did not believe the principles applied to themselves. They associated the code with Nazi atrocities such as systematic murder and torture, but they could not see how such a code could apply to them. Indeed some of the American medical community either "claimed ignorance of the document or ignored it" (9). For example, the first principle of the Code, that subjects "should have legal capacity to give consent…exercise free power of choice, without the element of force…constraint or coercion" would appear to preclude the inclusion of prisoners in any clinical research study, yet Hornblum cites a number of examples, post Nuremberg, where prisoners in the US, who were by definition not free of constraint, were used for clinical studies of histoplasmosis, infectious hepatitis, syphilis, and amoebic dysentery (9). Utilitarian principles seemed to prevail in the post-war United States and appeared to trump any consideration of the principles laid out in the Nuremberg Code. Similar abuses of informed consent were reported throughout the 1960s and 70s in the United States.

From 1963 a New York team deliberately infected the 'mentally retarded' with hepatitis at Willowbrook, an institution on Staten Island, so that experimental vaccines could be tested (10). As we have already learned in chapter 5, between 1932 and 1972 investigators from the US Public Health Service followed a group of Alabama farm workers in Tuskegee to learn about the natural history of syphilis (11). In the process, and to avoid disruption of their experiment, they denied the men the benefits of penicillin therapy and subjected them to various investigations including lumbar punctures, which they passed off as treatments for so-called 'bad blood'. In the early 1960s a team at the Jewish Chronic Disease Hospital in Brooklyn, injected live cancer cells into elderly, debilitated cancer patients without their consent (12).

In conducting such experiments the physicians involved were directly contradicting the principles outlined in the Nuremberg Code. This may be taken as evidence that those American physicians felt the code only applied to the Nazis who were involved in mass murder and torture and not to honest American doctors who would always act in the best interest of their patients according to the Hippocratic oath.

CODES OF PRACTICE BEFORE NUREMBERG

While the Nuremberg Code is undoubtedly the most well known code of practice for clinical trials, and one that has been used as the prototype for future codes including those which we use today, it was not the first, nor even the first to have its origins in Germany.

In 1898, Albert Neisser, an eminent German physician, conducted a number of experiments investigating serum therapy in patients with syphilis (13). In an attempt to vaccinate healthy individuals against syphilis he injected them without their knowledge or consent with serum from syphilis sufferers. Some of these subjects contracted the disease and Neisser concluded the "vaccination" did not work. This case was discussed in the press and by the Prussian parliament and in 1899 they asked the government to act. Neisser was fined and in 1900 the Minister for Religious, Education and Medical Affairs issued a directive to all hospitals and clinics, which stated that if "the human subject was a minor or not competent for other reasons" all medical interventions were to be strictly excluded other than for diagnosis, healing or immunisation (13). The Directive went on to state that the subject must give their "unambiguous consent" after a "proper explanation of the possible negative consequences" of the intervention. All research interventions could be performed only by the medical director or with their authorisation. In all cases, fulfilment of these requirements as well as further circumstances of the case had to be "documented in the medical history".

This directive, which is known as the Berlin or Prussian Code of 1900, was not, however, legally binding, but in 1931 Germany introduced a number of regulations to protect human research subjects which were. This Reichsrundschreiben document entitled "Regulations on New Therapy and Human Experimentation" did become legally binding in Germany, between 1931 and 1945. Paradoxically, then, Germany during the Second World War was the only country with legally binding and ethically advanced guidelines on human experimentation (14). However, the existence of this legal framework did not prevent the atrocities of medical experimentation that were revealed at Nuremberg.

The Reichsrundschreiben contained 14 points and guidelines that follow on from, and elaborate on, the Hippocratic tradition (15). They state that consent of the individual is required for experiments involving "innovative therapies" and also human experimentation. For human experimentation an informed consent was required except in urgent cases where the subject's life needed saved or if serious harm was to come to the subject (15). Concerning Human Experimentation, consent was therefore absolutely essential. Also the use of children was only acceptable if there was no risk of harm and experimentation on the terminally ill was completely forbidden (15).

Conclusion

What history teaches us here is very clear. Having a code of ethical practice for experimentation on humans, even if ratified by law is no insurance against atrocity. This should lead us to question the validity of codes of practice *per se*. Their existence is one thing; our adherence to them is quite another. If Buchenwald and Ravensbrück can happen in a country regulated by a legal framework demanding the informed consent of subjects in clinical research; if Willowbrook and Tuskegee can happen in a country whose leading physicians drafted the Nuremberg Code, what purpose do such codes fulfil?

Any code of practice, whether voluntary or statutory, will only be effective if individual practitioners consider that it applies to them. Clearly, the Nazi physicians paid no heed to their own laws for they did not believe that the inmates of concentration camps were covered by such legislation. In his opening remarks at the Doctors' Trial Taylor stated, "To their murderers these wretched people were not individuals at all" (2). Perhaps this surrendering of individuality, this perceived loss of humanity allowed the Nazi physicians to justify their actions. But what of the many other examples of misconduct and atrocity that have occurred since Nuremberg? Again, we may be dealing with investigators who for one reason or another feel that the codes of practice do not apply to them or their particular form of experimentation. Perhaps they have even lost sight of the humanity of their trial subjects. We must understand and fully accept the consequences of our actions in any clinical trial setting. While codes of practice give us a framework for our actions, ultimately they will be redundant if we do not, as individual practitioners, learn about them, understand them and, of course, follow them. In the UK, and throughout Europe the most recent step-change in the regulation of clinical trials was imposed by the implementation of the European Union Directive on Clinical Trials (16). This new legislation was introduced into the UK in 2004 as the Medicines for Human Use (Clinical Trials) Regulations (17) and makes it compulsory to conduct human clinical trials of investigational medicinal products in accordance with the principles and conditions of Good Clinical Practice. These principles include adherence to strict ethical standards many of which can be traced directly back to the Nuremberg Code. Since its introduction this legislation has prompted considerable disquiet amongst clinical researchers, largely because of the additional administrative burdens placed upon them (18). However, if we need to remind ourselves why such codes of practice are required we only need to glance backwards in history. The complexity of modern codes is, however, a cause for concern. While we may as clinical researchers agree with them in principle and be more than willing to adhere to them, if such codes are seen as presenting obstacles to research without adding to patient safety, then they will be ignored. Codes of practice have been ignored before; to prevent it happening again we, as a research community, must ensure that their relevance and practicality is as much a consideration in their drafting as the ethical ideals which they hope to serve.

REFERENCES

1. Anonymous. The brutality of Nazi physicians [Editorial]. *Journal of the American Medical Association* 1946; 132:714
2. United States v Karl Brandt et al. Trials of War Criminals (T. Taylor, opening statement of the prosecution). Washington DC: Government Printing Office, 1949

70

3. Lifton RJ. The Nazi doctors: medical killing and the psychology of genocide. Basic Books, 1988.
4. United States v Karl Brandt et al. Trials of War Criminals. Washington DC: Government Printing Office, 1949: 9114–228
5. The Nuremberg Code [from *Trials of War Criminals before the Nuremberg Military Tribunals under Control Council Law No. 10*. Nuremberg, October 1946–April 1949. Washington, D.C.: U.S. G.P.O, 1949–1953.] http://www.ushmm.org/research/doctors/Nuremberg_Code.htm (Accessed May 08, 2009.
6. Shuster E. The Nuremberg Code: Hippocratic ethics and human rights. *Lancet* 1998; 351: 974-7.
7. Shevell MI. Neurology's witness to history: Part II: Leo Alexander's contributions to the Nuremberg Code (1946 to 1947) *Neurology* 1998; 50:274-8.
8. Temme LA, Ethics in human experimentation: the two military physicians who helped develop the Nuremberg Code. *Aviation Space and Environmental Medicine* 2003; 74:1297-300.
9. Hornblum AM. They were cheap and available: prisoners as research subjects in twentieth century America. *British Medical Journal* 1997; 315: 1437–41
10. Moreno JD, Lederer SE. Revising the history of cold war research ethics. *Kennedy Institute of Ethics Journal* 1996; 6: 223–38
11. US Public Health Service. Final Report of the Tuskegee Syphilis Study Ad Hoc Advisory Panel. Washington DC: US Department of Health, Education, and Welfare, Public Health Service,1973
12. Beecher HK. Ethics and clinical research. *New England Journal of Medicine* 1966; 274: 1354–60

13. Vollmann, J, Winau R. Informed consent in human experimentation before the Nuremberg code. *British Medical Journal* 1996; 313: 1445-7.
14. Principles of Research in Human Subjects http://www.gwu.edu/~nsarchiv/radiation/dir/mst reet/commeet/meet2/brief2/tab_i/br2i1d.txt (Accessed May 8, 2009)
15. Sass HM. Reichsrundschreiben 1931: Pre-Nuremberg German regulations concerning new therapy and human experimentation. *Journal of Medical Philosophy* 1983; 8: 99-111.
16. Directive 2001/20/EC of the European Parliament and of the Council of 4 April 2001 on the approximation of the laws, regulations and administrative provisions of the Member States relating to the implementation of good clinical practice in the conduct of clinical trials on medicinal products for human use. *Official Journal of the European Communities* 2001; L121: 34-44.
17. Statutory Instrument 2004 No. 1031 The Medicines for Human Use (Clinical Trials) Regulations 2004. http://www.hmso.gov.uk/si/si2004/20041031.htm (Accessed May 8, 2009)
18. Griffin GE, Brown M, Gilmore I et al. UK research trials are on verge of extinction. [Letter] *The Times* January 14, 2009.

GLOSSARY OF TERMS AND ABBREVIATIONS

Like many areas of medicine, the field of clinical trials is awash with abbreviations and acronyms. Whether you are coming to this topic for the first time or are a seasoned trialist you may encounter terms and abbreviations that are unfamiliar. The following list is far from exhaustive but may be of use if you wish to read further.

ABPI	Association of the British Pharmaceutical Industry
ADR	Adverse Drug Reaction
AE	Adverse Event
AHP	Authorised Health Professional
BMA	British Medical Association
BNF	British National Formulary
BP	British Pharmacopoeia
BSI	British Standards Institution
CDC	Center for Disease Control & Prevention (US)
CFR	US Code of Federal Regulations (US)
CI	Chief Investigator
CRA	Clinical Research Associate or Assistant
CRF	Case Record/Report Form
CRO	Contract Research Organisation/Clinical Research Officer
CSM	Committee on Safety of Medicines
CT	Clinical Trial
CTA	Clinical Trial Authorisation
CTIMP	Clinical Trial of Investigational Medicinal Product
DSMB	Data Safety Monitoring Board
e-CRF	Electronic Case Report (or record) Form

EMEA	European Medicines Evaluation Agency
EU	European Union
EUDRA	European Union Drug Regulatory Authorities
EUDRACT	European Clinical Trials Database
FDA	Food and Drug Administration (US)
FTIM	First Time in Man
GCP	Good Clinical Practice
GDP	Good Distribution Practice
GLP	Good Laboratory Practice
GMC	General Medical Council
GMP	Good Manufacturing Practice
GP	General Practitioner
HMO	Health Maintenance Organisation (US)
ICD	International Classification of Diseases
ICH	International Conference on Harmonisation
ICH-GCP	International Conference on Harmonisation – Good Clinical Practice
IEC	Independent Ethics Committee
IMP	Investigational Medicinal Product
IRAS	Integrated Research Application System
IRB	Institutional Review Board (outside the U.S referred to as Independent Ethics Committees)
MedDRA	Medical Dictionary for Regulatory Activities
MHRA	Medicines and Healthcare products Regulatory Agency
MRC	Medical Research Council
MREC	Main Research Ethics Committee
NHS	National Health Service
NICE	National Institute for Clinical Excellence (UK)

NRES	National Research Ethics Service
OTC	Over the Counter
Phase I	Initial Clinical Trials in patients to test drug safety
Phase II	Clinical Trials in patients to test drug efficacy
Phase III	Clinical trials in patients for additional safety, efficacy, & other information
Phase IV	Clinical Trials after drug marketed, surveillance studies
PI	Principal Investigator
QA	Quality Assurance
QC	Quality Control
R&D	Research & Development
RCT	Randomised Controlled Trial
REC	Research Ethics Committee
SAE	Serious Adverse Event
SDV	Source Data Verification
SE	Standard Error
SEM	Standard Error of Mean
SI	Statutory Instrument
SMO	Site Management Organisation
SOP	Standard Operating Procedure
SUSAR	Suspected Unexpected Serious Adverse Reaction
TMF	Trial Master File
WHO	World Health Organization
WMA	World Medical Association

WEB RESOURCES

This is a list of websites that provide information related to clinical trials. There are a number of sites relating to the UK legislative framework, but also more general resources. Websites are arranged under the following headings:

1. UK clinical trials legislation
2. Other related UK Legislation
3. General Information - Clinical Trials
4. General Information - Drug Development & EU
5. Research Quality
6. Ethics and Informed Consent
7. US Legislation & Regulatory Bodies

All websites were accessed on January 5th 2009.

I.   UK clinical trials legislation

www.nres.npsa.nhs.uk
National Research Ethics Service (NRES). The organisation responsible for co-ordinating ethics committees in the UK. From this site you may obtain the electronic ethics committee application form and guidance on obtaining ethical approval for all NHS related research, including clinical trials.

www.ct-toolkit.ac.uk/
This is a useful site for guidance on the practical implementation of the EU Directive and the Medicines for Human Use legislation in the UK, particularly for non-commercially funded research. It provides access to a wide range of relevant documents including forms, guidance documents and related materials. It has been created by the Department of Health/Medical Research Council joint working groups that

were set up to advise on the implementation of the Clinical Trials Directive.

www.emea.europa.eu/
The European Agency for the Evaluation of Medicinal Products (EMEA) – This body was established by Council Regulation EEC 2309/93 of 22 July 1993. It co-ordinates and supports the EU licensing system.

eudract.emea.europa.eu/
This website provides access to the EudraCT system where you may register a clinical trial and obtain supporting documentation.

eudravigilance.emea.europa.eu/highres.htm
This also allows access to the EudraVigilance guidance.

www.mhra.gov.uk/index.htm
This is the official site of the Medicines and Healthcare Products Regulatory Agency (MHRA). This is the executive agency of the Department of Health, controlling medicines, healthcare products and medical equipment. It was formed from a merger of the Medicines Control Agency (MCA) and the Medical Devices Agency (MDA) on 1 April 2003.

www.mhra.gov.uk/home/groups/comms-ic/documents/publication/con007544.pdf
A useful 19-page reference entitled *A Guide to what is a medicinal product* which has been produced by the MHRA to help clarify this sometimes thorny issue.

www.opsi.gov.uk/si/si2004/20041031.htm
Medicines for Human Use (Clinical Trials) Regulations 2004. The statutory instrument which transposes the EU Clinical

Trials Directive into UK law. This was laid before parliament on 1ˢᵗ April, 2004.

www.opsi.gov.uk/si/si2006/uksi_20061928_en.pdf
2006 No. 1928 Amendment to Medicines for Human Use (Clinical Trials) Regulations 2004. The first amendment to Statutory Instrument No. 1031

www.opsi.gov.uk/si/si2006/uksi_20062984_en.pdf
2006 No. 2984 Amendment to Medicines for Human Use (Clinical Trials) Regulations 2004. The second amendment to Statutory Instrument No. 1031

www.opsi.gov.uk/si/si2008/pdf/uksi_20080941_en.pdf
2008 No. 941 Amendment to Medicines for Human Use (Clinical Trials) Regulations 2004. The third amendment to Statutory Instrument No. 1031

www.eortc.be/Services/Doc/clinical-EU-directive-04-April-01.pdf
Text of the EU Clinical Trials Directive (2001/20/EC).

europa.eu.int/eur-lex/lex/LexUriServ/site/en/oj/2005/l_091/l_09120050409 en00130019.pdf
Text of the EU GCP directive (2005/28/EC) which clarifies what is required in order to conduct a clinical trial in accordance with Good Clinical Practice.

www.ich.org/cache/compo/276-254-1.html
Text of the ICH Good Clinical Practice Guidelines can be found using the side menus going through Guidelines / Efficacy / Good Clinical Practice

pharmacos.eudra.org/F2/pharmacos/dir200120ec.htm
EU commission site to access all the guidance documents for the implementation of Directive 2001/20/EC.

www.tmn.ac.uk/
The UK Trial Managers' Network (UKTMN) is a forum for those running publicly-funded trials. Its primary functions are to link trial managers together to ensure the sharing and dissemination of expertise and experience and to provide training tools developed by the members of the network to new trial managers.

www.wma.net/e/policy/b3.htm
The Declaration of Helsinki, which was first published in 1964 and has been updated frequently since.

2. Other related UK Legislation

www.opsi.gov.uk/
Office of Public Sector Information, which now includes Her Majesty's Stationery Office (HMSO) online. This provides access to UK legislation.

www.opsi.gov.uk/acts/acts1990/Ukpga_19900023_en_1.htm
Access to Health Records Act, 1990 (c.23)

www.opsi.gov.uk/acts/acts1990/Ukpga_19900018_en_1.htm
The Computer Misuse Act, 1990

www.opsi.gov.uk/acts/acts1998/19980029.htm
The Data Protection Act, 1998

www.opsi.gov.uk/acts/acts1998/19980042.htm
The Human Rights Act, 1998

www.opsi.gov.uk/legislation/scotland/acts2000/20000004.htm
The Adults with Incapacity (Scotland) Act 2000. Part 5 deals with medical treatment and research.

www.opsi.gov.uk/acts/acts2000/20000023.htm
Regulation of Investigatory Powers Act, 2000

www.opsi.gov.uk/legislation/scotland/acts2000/20000011.htm
Regulation of Investigatory Powers (Scotland) Act, 2000

www.opsi.gov.uk/acts/acts2004/20040030.htm
Human Tissue Act 2004

www.show.scot.nhs.uk/confidentiality/publications/6074 NHSCode.pdf
NHS Code of Practice on Protecting Patient Confidentiality. Includes guidance on the requirements of the Data Protection Act, patient consent for use of their information and anonymisation.

www.sehd.scot.nhs.uk/cso/
Scottish Executive Health Department website where the publications section provides a copy of Research Governance Framework for Health and Community Care

3. General Information - Clinical Trials

www.actmagazine.com/appliedclinicaltrials/
Website of the *Applied Clinical Trials* journal, which provides a forum for the pharmaceutical industry and medical researchers.

clinicaltrials.gov/
A service of the US National Institutes of Health, developed by the National Library of Medicine. It provides a free trial registration site plus general information on the purpose of clinical trials and recruitment.

www.controlled-trials.com/mrct/mrct_about.asp
The *meta*Register of Controlled Trials (*m*RCT) is a major international searchable database of ongoing randomised controlled trials in all areas of healthcare, built by combining registers held by public, charitable and commercial sponsors of trials. It is a free service that allows users to search all participating registers and meets the requirements of the International Committee of Medical Journal Editors (ICMJC) for registration of clinical trials.

www.jameslindlibrary.org
A site managed by the Royal College of Physicians Edinburgh and an invaluable resource for the study of the history of medicine. This site includes articles and commentaries on many aspects of medical history and often includes pdfs of key original historical works that would be difficult to source in many libraries.

4. General Information - Drug Development & the EU

eur-lex.europa.eu/en/index.htm
Site for searching for html versions of EU legislation, including legislation in preparation.

www.ich.org/
International Conference on Harmonization (ICH) – Official Web site.

heads.medagencies.org/
The European Heads of Agencies (EEC-MRFG) web site lists all European medicines regulatory agencies and links to their sites.

5. Research Quality

www.barqa.com/
British Association of Research Quality Assurance – assuring good scientific practice in research and development.

www.diahome.org/DIAHome/
The Drug Information Association (DIA) was founded in the USA in 1964 as a non-profit, scientific association of professionals employed in academia and the pharmaceutical industry. It publishes the quarterly *Drug Information Journal.*

www.efgcp.be/
European Forum for Good Clinical Practice (EFGCP). This is a European 'think tank' for considering the ethical, regulatory, and scientific framework of clinical research.

www.nice.org.uk/
NICE - The National Institute for Clinical Excellence - was set up as a Special Health Authority for England and Wales. It is part of the National Health Service (NHS), and its role is to provide patients, health professionals and the public with authoritative, robust and reliable guidance on current "best practice".

www.rdforum.nhs.uk/
A network for those involved in planning and managing research in health and social care. Membership of the Forum is open to anyone involved, or interested, in managing and

planning research in the NHS or social care. Joining the Forum ensures that you receive regular e-mail newsletters.

6. Ethics and Informed Consent

www.myresearchproject.org.uk
IRAS - Integrated Research Application System. Streamline application form for submission of applications to several systems for approvals to conduct a clinical trial. This is part of the UKCRC work to streamline the approvals process.

www.nres.npsa.nhs.uk/
NRES guidance on Informed Consent and template for patient information sheet and consent forms.

www.dh.gov.uk/PolicyAndGuidance/HealthAndSocialCar eTopics/Consent/fs/en
UK Department of Health site providing information and guidance on obtaining consent from patients, for treatment or research.

www.wma.net/e/
The World Medical Association (WMA) is an international organization representing physicians. It was founded in 1947, to work for the highest possible standards of ethical behaviour and care by physicians. It has been responsible for a number of ethical guidelines including the Declaration of Helsinki

7.   US Legislation & Regulatory Bodies

www.access.gpo.gov/index.html
US Government Printing Office Site – Searchable site listing entire Code of Federal Regulations (CFR) including title 21 (Food and Drugs).

www.access.gpo.gov/nara/cfr/waisidx_98/21cfr312_98.ht ml
21 CFR 312 Investigational New Drug Regulations

www.fda.gov/cder/
Home page for the Center for Drug Evaluation & Research (CDER). This is part of the FDA that deals with new drug applications.

www.fda.gov/default.htm
Home page of the Food & Drugs Administration (FDA), which is the US public health agency responsible for overseeing human and veterinary drugs, biological products, medical devices, the nation's food supply, cosmetics, and products that emit radiation.

SUGGESTIONS FOR FURTHER READING

Hopefully, after you have read this book, you may be stimulated to read more on the topics discussed here. There are, however, more books written about clinical research, medical ethics and the history of medicine than it is possible to read in a reasonable lifetime. So where should you begin? Below I have listed some of the many books which you may find interesting. Should you wish to obtain any of these suggested texts you will find them by searching on Amazon. Alternatively, you will find them all listed separately at the Amazon Bookstore on my website www.allangaw.com

Annas J and Grodin MA (eds) (1995) The Nazi Doctors and the Nuremberg Code: Human Rights in Human Experimentation, OUP USA.

> [A multi-author book containing a wealth of useful material and commentary on the development of the Nuremberg Code.]

Franklin B (2008) Autobiography and Other Writings (Oxford World's Classics), Oxford Paperbacks.

> [Franklin, the founding father, the statesman, but also the inventor and scientist, are revealed in his own words which have never been out of print since he wrote them.]

Furberg BD and Furberg CD (2007) Evaluating Clinical Research: All That Glitters Is Not Gold (2nd Ed), Springer.

> [A wealth of insight, served up with a collection of witty cartoons, makes what could have been a dry subject more than palatable.]

Gallin J (2007) Principles and Practice of Clinical Research (2nd Edn), Academic Press; 2 edition

> [One of the better multi-author textbooks on clinical trials. It has an opening chapter on the history of clinical trials but the remainder is probably of most use to a potential investigator – bear in mind, however, it is written with a US focus.]

Gregory W (2005) Animal Magnetism; or, Mesmerism and Its Phenomena, Adamant Media Corporation.

> [A facsimile reprint of a book from 1877 written by a later advocate of animal magnetism. Interesting from an historical perspective.]

Jones JH (1992) Bad Blood: The Tuskegee Syphilis Experiment (2nd Edn), The Free Press.

> [A thorough and exhaustive exposition and undeniably the definitive work on the subject.]

Lifton RJ (1988) The Nazi Doctors: Medical Killing and the Psychology of Genocide, Basic Books.

> [A large and painstakingly researched book which goes further than most books of this genre in examining the thought processes of the Nazi medical personnel.]

Mesmer FA (2002) Magnétisme animal. Mémoires et aphorismes de Mesmer, Adamant Media Corporation.

> [If your French is up to it, this is the original from Mesmer himself.]

Pagel W (2002) Joan Baptista Van Helmont: Reformer of Science and Medicine (Cambridge Studies in the History of Medicine) Cambridge University Press.

> [A detailed biography of Van Helmont which covers his life and many works, focussing principally on his work in the field of chemistry.]

Pocock S (1983) Clinical Trials: A Practical Approach (Wiley Medical Publications), Wiley Blackwell.

> [The author is a renowned statistician and his approach is both practical and highly readable.]

Schmidt U (2004) Justice at Nuremberg: Leo Alexander and the Nazi Doctors' Trial, Palgrave Macmillan.

> [As the title suggests this focuses on the part played by the American physician Leo Alexander at the Nuremberg Trial and his part in the development of the Nuremberg Code.]

Schmidt U (2007) Karl Brandt - The Nazi Doctor: Medicine and Power in the Third Reich, Hambledon Continuum.

> [Schmidt's second book – this time focussing on Hitler's personal physician and the most senior defendant at the Doctors' Trial in Nuremberg.]

Weindling PJ (2006) Nazi Medicine and the Nuremberg Trials: From Medical Warcrimes to Informed Consent, Palgrave Macmillan.

> [A very detailed exposition and analysis of the Doctors' Trial itself.]

INDEX

88